Dr Frank Tallis is an award-winning writer and clinical psychologist. He has held lecturing posts in clinical psychology and neuroscience at the Institute of Psychiatry and King's College London, and is one of the country's leading authorities on obsessional states. He is author of *Understanding Obsessions and Compulsions* (Sheldon Press), recommended on the Reading Well Books on Prescription scheme. He has written academic textbooks and over 30 academic papers in international journals, and psychology books for the general reader: *Changing Minds: A History of Psychotherapy as an Answer to Human Suffering, Hidden Minds: A History of the Unconscious, Love Sick: Love as a Mental Illness* and *The Incurable Romantic: and Other Unsettling Revelations*. In 1999 Frank Tallis received a Writers' Award from the Arts Council and in 2000 he won the New London Writers' Award. Frank Tallis' novels are: *Killing Time* (Penguin), *Sensing Others* (Penguin), *Mortal Mischief* (Arrow), *Vienna Blood* (Arrow), *Fatal Lies* (Arrow), *Darkness Rising* (Arrow), *Deadly Communion* (Arrow), *Death and the Maiden* (Arrow) and *Mephisto Waltz* (Pegasus). The novels have featured to much acclaim in several national and international literary awards.

Overcoming Common Problems Series

Selected titles

A full list of titles is available from Sheldon Press on our website at
www.sheldonpress.co.uk

Lists of titles in the Mindful Way and Sheldon Short Guides series are also available from Sheldon Press.

Overcoming Common Problems

How to Stop Worrying

Second edition

DR FRANK TALLIS

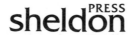

First published in 1990

This edition published by Sheldon Press in 2019
An imprint of John Murray Press
An Hachette UK company

1

A CIP catalogue record for this title is available from the British Library

Paperback ISBN 978 1 52932 922 3
eBook ISBN 978 1 84709 316 5

Typeset by Cenveo® Publisher Services
Printed and bound in Great Britain by Clays Ltd, Elcograf S.p.A.

John Murray Press policy is to use papers that are natural, renewable
and recyclable products and made from wood grown in sustainable forests.
The logging and manufacturing processes are expected to conform to the
environmental regulations of the country of origin.

Sheldon Press
Carmelite House
50 Victoria Embankment
London EC4Y 0DZ

www.sheldonpress.co.uk

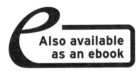

**Also available
as an ebook**

Contents

1

What is worry?

Let us start with an example.

Janet

Bob had told Janet that he would be home by seven. At five to seven, Janet noted the time, sat down and began to flick through a magazine. At 7.15, she looked at the clock again. Bob was usually punctual. She considered the time and decided that he must have been delayed; the train perhaps? She started to read an article, but found it difficult to concentrate. At the end of each column she noted the time. When she reached the end of the second page, she realized that although she had actually read all the words on the page, she couldn't remember any of it. Thoughts began to enter her head: 'I wonder why he's late? It's half-past seven now. He usually calls or texts me if anything's happened.' Janet put the magazine down and switched on the television. For a couple of minutes she was able to concentrate, but when she noticed it was twenty to eight she sent a quick text and then, when there was no reply, called Bob on his mobile. He didn't pick up. Janet got up and began to walk around the room. The thoughts had started again: 'If he knew about the delay he would have texted or called. He always does. Why didn't he answer his phone? I hope everything's all right. What if . . .' At this point Janet began to feel very uneasy, imagining the telephone ringing and somebody telling her sympathetically that Bob had been involved in an accident. At eight o'clock, she heard the key in the door, and sighed with relief when Bob came in cursing the railway system and the fact that his phone had run out of battery.

The above situation is fictional, but it represents a fairly typical example of worry. What, then, is worry? In spite of the fact that most people experience worry, professional mind-watchers like psychologists and psychiatrists have had very little to say about it. In fact, it is only over the past few years that worry has been given any serious consideration at all.

Although professionals have failed to provide us with an agreed definition of worry, this shouldn't deter us from attempting to describe it and establishing some common features of worry. Let us take another look at what happened to Janet during her worry episode.

The first thing is that Janet couldn't concentrate. Her attention was constantly being interrupted by thoughts about Bob. Not just any thoughts, but bad, uncontrollable ones. Janet would have saved herself from an extremely unpleasant hour waiting if she had only been able to read her magazine or watch television. However, her bad thoughts tended to get worse and worse, a process sometimes called 'catastrophizing'. Lack of control over repetitive bad thoughts and a tendency to think things are going to get worse are two important features of worry.

The idea that thoughts cannot be controlled during a worry episode is reflected in everyday speech. How often have you heard someone say, 'I'm a born worrier'? In other words, I was born like this and have no choice in the matter. It is, of course, true that some people seem to worry more than others. However, it is not true that if you appear to be a 'born worrier' you must remain one for the rest of your life. This book is about how you might learn to control your worries. We will not attempt to 'treat' or 'cure' worry, because this would be extremely unwise. As you are about to find out, in some situations worry might have some very real advantages.

Does worry have a purpose?

Thoughts and feelings don't just happen. They occur for a reason. Let's take a closer look at fear to illustrate this point. When you get frightened, certain things happen to your body. Chemicals, like adrenaline, are released into the blood, causing many changes to take place: an increase in heart rate, 'heavy' breathing, sweating and the movement of blood away from some areas of the body – for example the skin – to the muscles (making a frightened person look pale). This accounts for the use of common expressions like 'white as a sheet', to describe the blanched complexion of a person in fright.

These changes occur simply to prepare the body for action. The emotion of fear is associated with threat. When an individual is threatened, then he or she can do one of two things to cope with the situation: either run away or confront the problem 'head on'. These two responses are sometimes called 'flight' and 'fight'. The physical changes that occur during fear are those that equip us best for fight or flight. An increased heart rate, and the movement of blood away from areas like the skin, will supply the muscles with all the chemicals required for vigorous activity. In other words, the muscles can work more efficiently. Because of this increased efficiency, when frightened an individual will be able to fight 'harder' and run faster, depending of course on which response is chosen.

Fear, then, alters your body so that the chances of surviving a dangerous situation are improved. The idea that feelings have useful functions is not a new one. In fact, Charles Darwin, the famous originator of the theory of evolution, was the first person to suggest that certain characteristics appear in both humans and animals because they have helped the species to survive. Clearly, fear is an extremely helpful emotion, albeit unpleasant.

So, why do people worry and in what way is it useful? Although some people claim to worry over nothing, this is usually untrue. What they probably mean is that they worry about things that sound trivial to other people. Worry is a response to a problem. When people realize that things are not going well or a particular situation might end unpleasantly, they worry. For most people, this will be experienced as a series of intrusive thoughts and images that won't go away.

Perhaps worry acts like an internal alarm system, which is a good thing because if you fail to deal with a potentially bad situation immediately the alarm will carry on until you do. In addition, the increasing strength of the alarm will make it more and more difficult for you to ignore it.

Roger

Roger has just said something hurtful to his wife, Jackie. Although he knows that he is in the wrong, he finds it difficult to apologize. Initially, he is able to carry on as usual. However, he soon begins to feel apprehensive, thinking: 'I wonder if she'll talk to me tonight . . . probably not. I didn't think she'd take it that badly . . . I hope she doesn't decide to go out. What if she has decided to go over to her mother's? Maybe she'll stay there. Just for the night. On the other hand, she might stay longer. No . . . she wouldn't. But . . . she might. She was pretty upset. Maybe she was very upset. We haven't been getting on very well lately. Maybe she'll start wondering whether it's all worth it. Perhaps . . . perhaps I should apologize.'

In a short space of time, Roger is forced to do 'the right thing' because of the increasing intensity of his worries. You will remember the catastrophizing which we mentioned earlier. When people catastrophize, the thoughts and images that they experience become more and more distressing.

Another helpful effect of worry might be preparation. When treating people with phobias (or irrational fears), psychologists use a group of techniques involving *exposure*. For example, someone scared of spiders might be asked to sit next to a jar containing a spider. In other words, the person is 'exposed' to something that makes him or her frightened. At first, this will feel quite uncomfortable. However, after a while, this discomfort is likely to go away. Sometimes a psychologist might ask the person to imagine a spider before presenting a real one. Even simply imagining a spider for about half an hour can sometimes have the effect of reducing fear. Worry might work in a similar way. If thoughts and images relating to an unpleasant situation keep on coming into your mind, then this might help you to deal with the situation when it actually happens. Repeated 'exposures' may have the effect of making you less scared of the anticipated situation and therefore more able to deal with it.

From the above we can see that worrying, although unpleasant, is in fact a perfectly normal thing to do. Worry might act as an alarm, telling you that a problem needs to be dealt with, while at the same time preparing you to deal with that problem. Worry is only a bad thing when it either starts unnecessarily or carries on for too long. Why, then, do some people worry more than others? We will try to answer this question next.

Why do I worry so much?

Everybody is different. We all have different beliefs and expectations. Because of these differences, no two people will react identically given the same situation. Although they might look as though they're responding in the same way, we can safely say that their thoughts will not correspond exactly. A single situation might trigger worry in one person, but not in another. In our introductory example, Janet thinks that because Bob is late, he has probably had an accident. She fails to consider all the other possibilities. Another person, less prone to worry than Janet, might have considered an accident as only one of several factors likely to cause Bob's lateness. Given how unlikely a serious accident actually is, our non-worrier might well have concluded that a train delay was the most likely reason for Bob's absence and carried on reading or watching television. Clearly, people who worry a lot tend to take a negative view of things and expect the worst. Why some people have this attribute and others don't is an extremely difficult question to answer. Perhaps it is a habit acquired during childhood. How we think and behave is strongly influenced by the way our parents think and behave. Parents provide children with example behaviours that tend to be copied. If we grow up in a family where it is normal to 'expect the worst', then it is quite likely that we will grow up 'expecting the worst' too.

Imagine that you are a 7-year-old child. You are being taken to school by your mother, who is unfortunately a worrier. On the way, your mother drops some clothes in at the dry cleaner's. The man in the shop says to your mother that the clothes will be ready tomorrow. Your mother asks him if he is sure. He says that he is, but your mother doesn't look convinced. When you step outside, your mother looks up at the sky, which is grey, same as usual. 'Come on,' she says, 'It's about to rain. We'll get soaked.' When you get to the bus stop, your mother looks at her watch: 'If this bus doesn't come soon, we're going to be late.' Growing up involves learning about the world. If you hear your parents predicting the worst possible outcomes in every situation, you too are likely to pick up the habit. Children pick up many mannerisms and expressions from their parents. It is possible that a negative view of things can be counted among those habitual responses acquired through imitation.

Although the above scenario is very plausible, note that at this stage we can only speculate on the influence of parenting on personality development and worry. Parental influence is probably only one of many factors that can shape our attitudes and beliefs. Others might include, for example, distressing life experiences. If you have had a lot of 'bad luck', and things keep on going wrong for you, then it will be difficult for you to maintain a positive picture of the world.

Although we can't provide a full explanation of why some people start worrying more than others, we can attempt to explain why some people carry on worrying and find it difficult to stop.

Before we do this, let's remind ourselves how worry is triggered. A situation is thought to be threatening because it contains the possibility of one or more bad outcomes. Thoughts and images remind the individual that there is a problem that needs to be dealt with. If the individual fails to deal with the problem, worry will continue. But if the problem is dealt with, worry will stop. At worst, a few unpleasant thoughts might continue to be a nuisance before disappearing altogether. Situations that make us worry are problem situations. In a way, they should be treated like crossword puzzles or anagrams. If you're doing a puzzle of any kind, you have to think about it first.

Everyday problem-solving can be broken down into a number of stages. First, it is useful to define the problem. This means expressing whatever it is that's bothering you in a very specific way. For example, 'I can't pay my heating bill.' The second stage is to think up as many ways of dealing with the problem as possible: for example, 'I could get a loan' or 'I could do some extra overtime at work.' The third stage is to decide which of these 'strategies' is the best one. Finally, the last stage is to implement the best strategy. In other words, to actually do it! We will consider problem-solving in more detail later.

Worriers appear to be very good at defining problems but extremely bad at solving them. There are a number of reasons why this might be. However, research has shown that worriers tend to be slower than non-worriers when attempting to make a decision. This delay seems to stem from a reluctance to make decisions unless they are absolutely sure that they are doing the right thing. So, when presented with a problem, a worrier will take longer to decide what to do about it than a non-worrier. This inability to make a quick decision is experienced as 'uncertainty' or 'doubt'.

Emily and Charlotte

Let's compare the circumstances of two women, Emily and Charlotte. They are both 35 years of age, both pregnant, and both naturally concerned that 'the baby will be all right'. In addition, both are aware that, at 35, it might be wise to undergo amniocentesis in order to determine the health of the child before birth. After 12 weeks, a foetus will begin to shed cells into the amniotic fluid surrounding it in the womb. Amniocentesis involves taking a sample of amniotic fluid by passing a needle through the abdomen and into the womb. The cells in the fluid can be inspected for abnormalities, which if serious may lead the parents to decide to terminate (or abort) the pregnancy. Unfortunately, there is a slight risk that amniocentesis can cause adverse reactions, resulting in a miscarriage.

Emily is a great worrier. Although she wants the test done she is worried about having a miscarriage. She is uncomfortable with the idea that amniocentesis isn't 100 per cent safe. She wants to be absolutely sure that her actions won't result in the loss of a perfectly healthy foetus. Of course, this is an impossible demand. She puts off making an appointment, and worries continuously: 'If I don't have the test done, then there might be something wrong with the baby . . . I'm not sure I could cope with that . . . but I don't want to lose this one; not if it's OK. That would be terrible . . . and amniocentesis isn't always accurate. They must get it wrong sometimes. Is it worth it? But . . . what if there is something wrong. Do I really want to know?'

Finally, Emily decides that amniocentesis is appropriate. She doesn't have a miscarriage, and some months later has a perfectly healthy baby.

Charlotte is much more decisive. She recognizes the risks associated with amniocentesis, but decides that these risks are reasonable. She decides right from the very beginning that amniocentesis is appropriate. Because she has made an early decision, there is no 'dilemma' as such and consequently she experiences less worry.

The longer it takes you to deal with a problem, the longer you will worry about it. Sometimes just deciding on a course of action will help you to stop worrying. If you make a decision to act in one way rather than another then you have reduced the uncertainty of your future. Most people find 'being uncertain' difficult to tolerate. When you make a decision, you reduce levels of uncertainty and make a commitment in the direction of dealing with your problem. These factors help to reduce worry.

Let's take a closer look at what happens when worriers delay decision-making. Whenever we make a decision we evaluate the evidence for and against it. High worriers seem to have unrealistically high evidence expectations. They want to know exactly what is going to happen if they decide to do 'this' rather than 'that'. Clearly, every decision we make is associated to a greater or lesser extent with a risk. It is impossible to see into the future, so it is also impossible to be absolutely sure that we are doing the right thing. In most situations, there just isn't enough evidence around to confirm that our decision is the best one. However, worriers are uncomfortable with this fact of life. Their decisions are delayed, because they go over things again and again in an attempt to be sure that what they are about to do is absolutely right.

Jenny

Let's consider an everyday example of this characteristic prolonging of a worry episode. As Jenny is driving to work, she suddenly realizes that she has no idea where her passport is. This is unfortunate because she has arranged a holiday in two weeks' time. She begins to worry. 'I wonder where it is? I can't remember! It must be somewhere. I couldn't have lost it, could I?' After a few minutes, she begins to catastrophize: 'I won't be able to go. I've already asked for leave now. I can't tell my boss I've changed my mind.' Jenny will continue to worry until she defines the problem and makes a decision.

If she had made a simple decision earlier, things might have been different. In her situation there are two possibilities. The passport really has been lost, and a new one must be applied for, or it's at home 'somewhere' and all she needs to do is look for it. As with all decisions she cannot be absolutely certain either way. However, you don't have to be absolutely certain to make most decisions. If Jenny were a non-worrier, she would most probably accept that the passport is somewhere at home, and not give it another thought for the rest of the day. In other words, she accepts what evidence is available and then makes a decision based on that evidence.

If worriers were able to make swifter decisions by accepting less evidence, worry would stop earlier. As you can see, indecision feeds worry. The longer you spend deliberating over a problem, the longer you are likely to spend worrying about it. We will be taking a close look at how to improve decision-making skills in Chapter 3.

This relationship between problems, evidence requirements and worry is shown in Table 1.1. First, a problem causes worry. To stop worry the problem must be solved. Because worriers want to be certain that they are doing the right thing, they find it difficult to choose a way of dealing with the problem. None of the solutions will provide sufficient evidence to guarantee that the problem will be solved. The longer the worrier spends thinking about what to do, the longer the problem remains unsolved. And because it remains unsolved, it will continue to trigger worry.

Table 1.1 How unsolved problems keep worry going

The worrier becomes aware of a problem

↓

this causes worry

↓

a decision is needed to resolve the problem

↓

the worrier fails to choose an appropriate plan

. . . because there's never enough evidence available to guarantee that a particular plan is absolutely right

↓

the problem remains

↓

which leads to more worry

Why do worriers require more evidence to make decisions?

Although we cannot say for sure why worriers are slower at making decisions than non-worriers, we can make a few educated guesses. First, it is possible that worriers are physically different. Perhaps their brains are 'wired' differently, so that decision-making takes longer. However, although one study has shown that worriers can produce different 'brainwaves' compared to non-worriers, there isn't really much evidence to suggest that worriers' brains are that different from those of anybody else. A second possibility is that worriers take longer to make decisions because of upbringing. For example, if parents have very high expectations, and also express strong disapproval when mistakes are made, then this might produce an overcautious child. If mistakes become associated with 'bad consequences', like punishment for instance, then a child might grow up striving to be absolutely certain that a decision is 'right'. This is because being right all the time will be a sure way of avoiding mother and father's disapproval. This disapproval might be communicated by anything from an unpleasant facial expression to a dreaded time out! If a child is forced into this behaviour pattern frequently, then it is likely to become automatic. In other words, by the time the child reaches adulthood, he or she will respond cautiously without really thinking about it. When decisions need to be made, decision-making will be unnecessarily delayed. The worried adult will look for signs that tell him or her that a particular decision is absolutely right. As we have already noted, this degree of certainty might not be necessary. A failure to make a decision might simply prolong worry.

What do people worry about?

Research has shown that different 'worries' can be divided into groups, each sharing a common theme. Worry items volunteered by members of the public were selected for inclusion in a worry questionnaire (Table 1.2). As you can see, 25 common worries have been grouped together under five headings: (1) intimate relationships; (2) lack of confidence; (3) aimless future; (4) work incompetence; and (5) financial problems. These titles reflect difficulties in the most important areas of everyday life. Worry is commonly experienced when something is perceived as going wrong in domestic, social or work situations. Research into satisfaction and happiness has shown that a good relationship, a full social life and an enjoyable job are particularly important factors in maintaining happiness.

Table 1.2 A worry questionnaire

Relationships

I worry

- that I will lose close friends;
- that I am unattractive to the opposite sex;
- that my family will be angry with me or disapprove of something that I do;
- that I find it difficult to maintain a stable relationship;
- that I am not loved.

Lack of confidence

I worry

- that I cannot be assertive or express my opinions;
- that others will not approve of me;
- that I lack confidence;
- that I might make myself look stupid;
- that I feel insecure.

Aimless future

I worry

- that I'll never achieve my ambitions;
- that I haven't achieved much;
- that my future job prospects are not good;
- that life may have no purpose;
- that I have no concentration.

Work incompetence

I worry

- that I will be late for an appointment;
- that I leave work unfinished;
- that I make mistakes at work;
- that I don't work hard enough;
- that I will not keep my workload up to date.

Financial problems

I worry

- that my money will run out;
- that I am not able to afford things;
- that financial problems will restrict holidays and travel;
- that my living conditions are inadequate;
- that I can't afford to pay bills.

Clearly, circumstances must affect the content of our worry episodes. Having plenty of money does not make people any happier; however, it does appear to reduce the number of unpleasant events they experience. Clearly, for somebody quite well off, getting a parking ticket might be considered a minor inconvenience, whereas for somebody hard up it might be perceived as a major financial catastrophe. Nevertheless, the influence of circumstances is less important than you might think. We know this by looking at how much people worry about the different areas included in the questionnaire. If a person worries about one area of life, then he or she will tend to worry about most of the others. So, high worriers tend to bring their tendency to worry with them wherever they go. For example, a person worried about relationships is also likely to worry about his or her work situation. Similarly, a person worried about social contact is also likely to worry about lack of direction in life. These findings seem to show that worriers are in some way different from non-worriers. They have a distinguishing 'characteristic' that causes them to worry in any circumstance.

We have already suggested that worry fills up the time between realizing that there is a problem and solving that problem. Because problems occur in all areas of life, a failure to resolve these problems will produce frequent worry associated with all these areas.

In addition to the areas included on the questionnaire, another group of worries is often reported to do with health concerns, often anticipating serious illness or death. In this group we also find worries about accidents. However, these worries are not as common as those mentioned above. In addition, over-concern with one's health is commonly associated with more serious anxiety problems. As this book is about common or ordinary worry, we will not consider this group in too much detail, although health concerns will be considered briefly in Chapter 6.

How do I know if I'm worrying too much?

Earlier, it was suggested that worry is like an alarm system that tells you to deal with a specific problem. Therefore, you should try to see worry as a friend rather than a foe – helpful, not harmful.

However, if you find that worry leads to more worry instead of decisions and actions, you might consider what effect this is having on your health. Unnecessary worry is a stress you could probably do without.

Very few studies have looked at the effect of worry on health, though there is some evidence to suggest that too much worry *is* bad for you. For example, one study found that people who worried excessively about a fairly routine hospital operation took longer to recover afterwards. Although there are only a few studies like this one, it is still possible to suggest ways in which worry might be harmful by looking at research into stress.

Most people believe that worry can change both the way we physically feel and our appearance. This is reflected in the way we use the word 'worry' in everyday speech: for example, describing people as having a 'worried look', or saying that we are 'worried sick'. People even attribute going grey to 'too much worry'. The word is strongly associated with looking and feeling bad, presumably because over the years people have noticed a relationship between worry and illness. Why should such a relationship exist? There are in fact a number of ways in which worry might cause health problems.

One of the most important findings in recent years has been the role of worry in insomnia or sleeplessness. Research shows that one of the main reasons for a 'sleepless night' is worry. Losing sleep is of course in itself unpleasant. However, an irregular pattern of sleep may well disrupt the fragile balance of chemicals that keeps us healthy. Chemicals called hormones are released at different points of the day. For example, one called prolactin is released mostly during sleep. Disturbed sleep patterns might lead to hormone-level changes, which in turn make certain types of illness more likely – anything from the common cold to something more serious.

In addition, research into stress has shown that attempting to cope with stressful situations for too long can lead to high blood pressure, which is one of the factors that increase the likelihood of heart attack. Because worriers are indecisive, everyday problems are prolonged. This means that they have to attempt to cope with unpleasant situations for longer periods of time. Wrestling with a problem for a long time might lead to increased blood pressure and subsequent health risks.

If you are getting more illnesses than usual, then perhaps you are under stress. Are you worrying a lot as a consequence? If so, is it getting you anywhere? Are unwanted thoughts making it difficult for you to get to sleep at night? If so, then you should start to take a closer look at those thoughts. Are they telling you something? Do you need to deal with an outstanding problem? In the next chapter we shall consider how we might prepare ourselves for the task of dealing with the problems that cause everyday worry.

2

Preparing to solve your problems

In the next two chapters we are going to consider how worry might be managed. We will do this by learning how to solve the everyday problems that prompt us to worry in the first place. However, before we discuss the techniques that might help us to achieve this, it will be necessary to explain a few things first.

If you are going to be an effective problem-solver, then you are going to need some practice. So, the first section of this chapter explains how important practice is. After this, you will be introduced to the idea of learning a 'problem-solving package'. Although the step-by-step process of problem-solving will not be considered in detail until Chapter 3, it will be useful to know what a 'problem-solving package' actually is.

In the third section of this chapter, it will be suggested that developing a positive attitude towards worry will make it less distressing. If you see worry as helpful, then you are more likely to use it constructively. Finally, you will be encouraged to recognize the early warning signs associated with the beginning of a period of worry, so that it will be easier to stop yourself becoming overwhelmed by unpleasant thoughts and images.

Practising skills

We have established that when we worry we are in fact responding to a problem. Therefore, to stop worrying we have to do something about whatever it is that started us worrying in the first place. To solve problems efficiently, we have to develop problem-solving 'skills'. It will be useful at this point to clear up what we mean by the word 'skills'. When someone is described as being skilled, it usually means being able to do something very well. Unless he or she is one of those extremely rare people born with a special gift, we assume that the skill was acquired through practice.

Relaxing

Every day, most people do things which are only possible because they are well practised. However, many of these activities are not recognized as requiring a special 'skill'. For example, many people assume that relaxation is easy, something that happens effortlessly when we aren't experiencing stress. Although this might be true for some people, it most certainly isn't true for all people. For many, learning to relax is as difficult as learning to drive. Relaxation techniques have to be taught and then, most important of all, practised regularly. People who suffer from anxiety are often advised to attend anxiety management training groups, where they are taught how to use relaxation to control the unpleasant feelings associated with anxiety. We all get anxious or stressed sometimes. It is only on these occasions that we realize how difficult relaxation is. You might be feeling very tense, and say to yourself, 'Just relax', but nothing happens. That is because you haven't practised relaxing. Relaxation is used here as an example, so we won't deal with relaxation techniques. However, if you feel that you might benefit from relaxation training, there are many books, CDs, DVDs and YouTube videos that explain what relaxation training is and how it works.

Another common example of something that people assume doesn't need practice is dieting. Most people decide to go on a low-calorie diet without giving the matter very much thought. But without preparing carefully, dieting is very difficult. For example, it is usually a good idea to stock up with low-calorie snacks like fruit, and to empty the larder of tempting high-calorie snacks like biscuits. If you don't take this kind of precaution, it's easy to end up hungry with nothing to keep you going but a packet of chocolate biscuits! Good preparation will increase your chances of success. After planning a diet it is then necessary to 'practise' it. Like learning to drive, some attempts will be more successful than others. Breaking a diet isn't that serious if you recognize that dieting is a skill. Setbacks can be used to identify areas that need more practice.

Relaxing and dieting are typical of a number of things that are not recognized as skills. It is very common for people to explain their disappointments by blaming themselves. For example, 'I can't relax because I'm a tense person' or 'I'll never lose weight because I haven't got any willpower.' However, unless you've actually practised something again and again, it's impossible to do. If you wanted to learn how to play the piano, you wouldn't blame yourself for not being able to play a tune after sitting at the keyboard once! This is because playing the piano is widely recognized as a skill. Nobody expects to be able to play Beethoven's 'Moonlight Sonata' without practising it first! However, for some reason we think that things like relaxing and dieting can be achieved without practice. This attitude invariably leads to 'failures', which lead in turn to self-recrimination and self-blame. The advantage of recognizing that things like relaxation and dieting are skills is that you cannot blame yourself if you don't succeed. You can't attribute your 'failure' to some 'bad' or 'weak' personality trait. You can only really blame yourself for not practising.

So what has all this got to do with worry? You will remember that in Chapter 1 we said that worry is like an alarm system that tells you it's time to deal with a problem. Once again, the ability to solve everyday problems is one of those things we tend to think of as automatic. We describe some people as though they are naturally 'good' at solving their problems, and others as though they are naturally 'bad'. If you happen to be bad at it, then there's not a lot you can do! In fact, solving everyday problems is a skill that can be easily learnt, and you don't have to be particularly clever. Indeed, research has shown that there is little correspondence between 'cleverness' and an ability to deal with 'life problems'. Among these we can include everyday stressful events like getting things done on time, as well as more serious matters like divorce or moving house. This lack of correspondence between 'cleverness' and the ability to cope with life shouldn't really be very surprising. After all, why should there be such a relationship? Solving an anagram requires skills that are very different from those required to cope with a 'rocky' marriage. Skills that are used to solve problems are generally grouped together as 'problem-solving packages'.

What is a problem-solving package?

If you were on holiday and decided to go for a long walk, you wouldn't just set off. You would probably buy or download a map first. This would allow you to plan a good route and prevent you from getting lost. When we are presented with a common life problem we also need a map – that is, a rough guide to the stages of problem-solving to help us plan a sensible route, leading to our destination. In other words, we will 'arrive' at an answer. Our guide to problem-solving will resemble a map in other ways too. For example, a map shows many different ways to get to the same place. For somebody who likes pretty views, an exhausting but picturesque route over hilly ground might be preferable to a flat coastal walk. For someone who likes the sea, the opposite will be true. Solving everyday problems is like finding the best route on a map, the one that you are happiest with. Usually, there are a number to choose from.

Sometimes, if a map isn't available, you ask for directions. You might be told to 'Go to the crossroads and turn left. If you can ford the river, go straight across, but if not, turn right and walk down to the bridge.' Directions are a list of instructions that help you to find your way. Our problem-solving package is just the same – a useful set of instructions that will help you to arrive at an answer. You might find that the easiest way is blocked. The river might be swollen because of heavy rainfall! In this case, you will have to find another way. But there are usually alternative ways of dealing with a problem. A problem-solving package will help you to work out alternative routes. In a way, the whole of this book is a problem-solving package. However, the really important part of this 'package' will be detailed in Chapter 3.

Changing your attitude towards worry

As suggested earlier, worry can be viewed as helpful rather than harmful. Unfortunately, because worry is unpleasant we often treat it as a problem in itself. Although worry can be 'problematic' it isn't really the problem as such. The *real* problem is the situation or person that's bothering us in the first place. Worry isn't the only warning system the body has. Physical pain is another. Imagine what would happen to someone who was unable to feel pain (and there *are* people like this). Let us suppose this person developed appendicitis. How would he or she know? Removing the appendix is a fairly routine operation; however, in most cases, it is important to remove it as soon as possible. Pain tells us that something is wrong; it prompts us to go to the doctor, who also uses pain when making a diagnosis. Although we think of pain negatively, pain saves lives. It makes us act quickly so that the physical problem causing pain is treated early.

Worry is to the mind what pain is to the body. One of the first things you must learn to do is change your attitude to worry, and view it as a helpful mental response that reminds you to deal with a problem. It has to be unpleasant and repetitive, or you wouldn't take any notice of it. Imagine buying an expensive security alarm system that went off very quietly for five seconds. Would you feel secure? Of course not! Anybody could gain entry to your home and you wouldn't know. However, if the alarm system starts loudly and continues until switched off it will be extremely difficult to miss. You will probably hear it as soon as it goes off, giving you enough time to get out of the house and to a place of safety before a potentially dangerous intruder can find you. Worry allows you to avoid potentially dangerous 'situations', by reminding you to solve related problems as soon as possible. Everyday problems are like intruders We need worry to let us know they're coming so that we can take appropriate action. So, let's start thinking about worry as a useful mental event rather than a burden – something that we can all take advantage of.

Recognizing worry

Worry is an involuntary activity. You don't decide when it begins, and once it has begun it is very difficult to stop. At first, a few negative thoughts and images might go through your mind. Then, as they become linked together they tend to tell a kind of 'story' which involves you or people you care about. For example, you might be concerned about a dental appointment. You might imagine what it will be like, travelling on the bus to the surgery. You might then imagine the waiting room. Eventually the story will get to the point where you sit in the chair and the dentist asks you to open your mouth. Perhaps you then think of something very unpleasant. For example, you might imagine the dentist making a mistake and pain in your gum. Suddenly, you become aware that you have been worrying. The story has been working towards an unpleasant climax, and it is only then that you realize how preoccupied you have been.

Worry often starts 'telling' you things in a quiet voice, a bit like having the radio on while you're doing something else. Suddenly, an item that interests you might come on, and you start listening again. While you were busying yourself, you were perhaps only partially aware of the broadcast.

Because worry tends to 'creep up' on you, it's important to recognize it early on. There are two good reasons for this. First, it's quite easy to get upset by worry, without really being aware of what's happening. This can sometimes have unfortunate consequences. When something is going on at 'the back of our minds', it often changes the way we feel, and this can in turn alter the way we behave. When we feel upset without recognizing why, it's easy to interpret those feelings incorrectly. We might blame somebody else for making us upset, even though we were upset already. This often happens when people are very busy. For example, if you are concentrating on an important job, it's easier to 'block out' worry. However, this mental 'block' is a bit like a poorly constructed dam. Negative thoughts and images might still trickle through, making you feel tense. Let's take an example to illustrate the point.

Helen

Helen had an exam coming up. However, she couldn't get time off work in which to revise. Her day at work was particularly demanding. She was being asked to meet an unrealistic deadline. Although she was able to concentrate on the job in hand, she would occasionally think about the exam. Her thoughts were almost all negative, and she anticipated failure. She became more and more 'uptight', without once acknowledging her worries. When Helen arrived home, John, her husband, started to chat about his day. Helen wasn't feeling very receptive and soon became irritated by John's conversation. When he asked her what the problem was, she could only say she felt 'tense'.

If Helen had acknowledged her worries, then she might have been able to give John a more satisfactory answer. A less ambiguous statement like 'I'm really worried about my exam' would have been more helpful. This would have made it clear to John that he hadn't really done anything wrong, and it would have also introduced the idea for further discussion. Together, they might have been able to work out how Helen might cope with the problem of her revision more successfully. If we recognize that we are worried, then at last we can start to think seriously about dealing with the worry or, more accurately, the problem that's causing it.

The second reason why it's important to recognize worry early is that it tends to get worse. If you are able to catch it before it really gets going, it might be possible to avoid the feeling of being overwhelmed, by which time you will probably be too upset to deal with your problems in a constructive way. Try to turn your worry into constructive problem-solving at the earliest possible opportunity.

An important thing to remember is that everybody responds to worry differently. Although feeling tense is often a sign that there is something bothering you, you may not always respond with tension. You might find that worry has the effect of making you feel more depressed than usual. Everybody is different, so in a way you will have to behave like a detective. You need to know what your early warning signs are. A good way of doing this is to keep a diary. Note how you're feeling at different points in the day, and then see if you can find reasons for those feelings. For example, you might notice that you feel tearful after someone has been rude to you. Somewhere, at the back of your mind, thoughts like 'I can't cope with this' and 'I can't face that person any more' might be quietly ticking over. In other words, underneath your upset feelings, you are beginning to worry. The alarm system is telling you that something is wrong and needs to be dealt with. Don't wait for worry to be intrusive. Try to recognize what your worry is telling you at the earliest convenient moment.

Most people are fairly consistent, responding to problems with a particular group of thoughts and feelings. However, you may find that different types of worry are associated with different early warnings. Worrying about how you act in social situations might make you feel tense, whereas worrying about failures might make you feel sad. The advantage of knowing your early warning signs is that you can stop yourself from getting very upset. If you take control of the worry process early, you will not get overwhelmed. As we said in Chapter 1, the process of catastrophizing might leave you with a pretty bleak view of the future.

Let's stop here a moment and summarize. First, make sure that when you catch yourself worrying, you remind yourself that these thoughts are letting you know that a problem needs to be dealt with. In this respect, worry can be viewed as a very useful reaction. Next, try to sort out what's bothering you early on. At this stage you don't have to do a detailed analysis of the problem. Just recognize you're feeling upset for a reason, and then try to get at least a rough idea of what you're upset about. Lastly, consider whether you're up to sorting things out.

This last point is quite important. If you're coming home from work on a crowded train in the rush hour with a splitting headache, you're probably not going to be able to think straight. Recognize that in stressful situations *you're not at your best*, so put off problem-solving until you're feeling calmer and attempt to distract yourself. If this doesn't work, try to separate yourself from your worries. and pretend that worry is like a radio broadcast or film. Let it run its course, but don't get drawn into it. Perhaps you could note down on a piece of paper the gist of what's bothering you, then make a resolution that you will give these worries some serious thought at a more convenient time. Being too 'wound-up' will affect your ability to solve problems. Perhaps after a hot relaxing bath your worries won't seem half as bad.

If you are feeling all right, then you're ready for the first stage of problem-solving – 'problem definition'. In the next chapter we will take a close look at defining problems and how to work out the best ways of dealing with them.

3

How to solve your problems:
the problem-solving package

Defining the problem

Defining a problem is surprisingly difficult. Worry will tell you where there is a problem, but it won't necessarily tell you the exact nature of the problem. Everyday problems can be extremely complex. Like an onion, they may have different layers that can be peeled away. Let's take an example.

Laura

Laura was worried about her workload. Although she was working very hard, she kept on making mistakes and had to do the same thing over and over again. She began to wonder what her boss would think of her and started to worry seriously about losing her job. She recognized that something should be done, but wasn't sure what. One of her ideas was to improve her work skills by doing a relevant evening class. Unfortunately, Laura had defined the problem in terms of her own inadequacy, an inaccurate definition. If we peel off a layer and look underneath, we find the true source of the problem – her new manager. Donald had been overfamiliar from the moment he arrived. Although he presented himself as a helpful sort of person, he punctuated his advice with tedious amorous advances. Now, Donald's comments were beginning to get Laura down. She had stopped going to Donald for advice, and consequently she was making some quite serious mistakes.

If Laura decides to attend evening classes, she might well improve her performance at work. However, this will not help in the long run. Donald will still have to be dealt with at some time. When you begin to worry about something, always look at your worry in context. A problem like Laura's – making mistakes every day – can be related to a bigger problem like sexual harassment. Because making mistakes happens more often, and has more immediate consequences, it is easy to forget that these mistakes are only happening *because* of the bigger problem.

Always think carefully about what is bothering you. A good way to find out is to talk things over with a friend. There's good evidence to suggest that the more you do this the better you feel. Perhaps discussing things helps people 'get to the bottom' of what's troubling them. In other words, they are able to define their problem more accurately, which in turn helps them to deal with it more effectively when the time comes.

Ben

Not all problems have different layers. Some are very simple. Let's take a look at a straightforward example for the sake of balance. Ben was worried about paying his gas bill. He knew that he had a cheque coming in the post, but was concerned that he would get cut off before it arrived. In Ben's case, the problem is not related to a bigger one. The gas company want some money. The answer is clearly to give them some. Ben rings them up, explains the situation and asks them to accept a temporary part-payment.

Although Laura's problem is complicated, and Ben's problem is straightforward, both of them have only *one* problem. Life is rarely that simple. You might well be worried about more than one thing, so you will have to define several problems. Try to see where one problem ends and another begins. You can do this by making a list; when your worries are written down, it's easier to see if they are connected. If your problems are unconnected, each will require special attention.

Don't attempt to solve all your problems at once. The best thing to do is take them one at a time. This means that you will have to put some worries on hold. This is going to be difficult, as the whole purpose of worry seems to be to capture your attention. However, as we said earlier, you can remind yourself that you are only delaying the solution of some problems as a temporary measure. You will of course deal with them as soon as you can. In addition to this, don't forget that by postponing addressing some problems, you will be able to deal with others more efficiently. You will really be able to concentrate on the problem in hand. By the time you get around to dealing with postponed problems, you should be less stressed, having disposed of others already.

We also mentioned distraction earlier. If you think you are likely to spend a whole evening worrying about problems that you intend to deal with but can't at present, then arrange to go out. An exciting film, or dinner with friends, might take your mind off things. Provided you are doing something about at least one of your problems, then you can afford to leave the others alone for a short while. However, don't forget that worry cannot really be ignored; distracting yourself can only ever be a 'stopgap' measure. Eventually, each problem will have to be dealt with, or worry will continue.

Until you are an accomplished problem-solver, it might be a good idea to start by attempting to solve your easiest problems first. Choose one that you can actually do something about. There are some things in life that you simply can't change. For example, if you have to go into hospital to have an operation, there's not a lot you can do about it. We will have more to say about this kind of problem in Chapter 6. Only attempt to solve problems that you have a sporting chance of solving.

Thinking up solutions (brainstorming)

After defining the source of your worry, the next thing to do is to ask yourself, 'What can I do about it?' Usually, if you are presented with a problem, it is possible to think of more than one answer. These answers are sometimes called 'coping strategies', because they represent ways of coping with the problem. The process of thinking up as many ways of dealing with a problem as possible is sometimes called 'brainstorming'.

You might ask at this point: why think up five ways of coping with a problem when one will do? The answer is to give yourself a choice. The more choice you have, then the more chance you have of selecting a way of coping that is just right for you. In addition, you might choose a particular way of coping because it looks good 'on paper', but when you actually try it out you may find it involves more than you bargained for. If you have thought up a number of different ways of dealing with a problem, all you have to do then is choose another. The basic idea of brainstorming is that quantity breeds quality. The more ideas you have, the more likely it is that one of them will be a really good one.

Before you start brainstorming there are a couple of things you should try to remember. The first is to suspend judgement. What this means is: don't be too self-critical. If you think up a way of dealing with a problem, then make a note of it, whatever it is. We can sort out the good ideas from the bad ones later. At this stage, the important thing is to stop yourself from dismissing ideas before you've given them a fair chance. Many people lack confidence in their own ability to cope with problems. Writing down as many ideas as you can will help you to get over a self-confidence barrier.

The second thing to remember before brainstorming is: don't be frightened to let yourself go! However farfetched some of your ideas might seem, write them down anyway. If you write down that you could deal with a financial problem by robbing a bank, then so be it. Clearly there will be some serious drawbacks to such a solution (drawbacks are considered in the next section). However, for the present, if you think up wild solutions then go ahead and write them down.

Many people have a tendency to say 'Yes, but . . .' when presented with a possible solution. One of the good things about brainstorming is that it will help you to overcome this tendency. If you say 'Yes, but . . .' too soon, you will never get the chance to evaluate your ideas fully. An incidental point to remember is that we are all sometimes reluctant to deal with our problems. After all, dealing with a problem often involves effort and, under some circumstances, confrontation. It might seem easier in the short term to avoid a particular problem than to deal with it. However, most problems don't solve themselves, and as long as we are aware of them they are likely to be a source of nagging worry. Let's take another example.

June

June had been a housewife since getting married 15 years previously. She felt so unfulfilled at home that this was making her depressed. She had begun to worry about the future. When her husband suggested that she might get a part-time job, her first reaction was 'Yes, but I'm not qualified to do anything.' She carried on thinking like this until a friend in a similar position got a job at a local play-centre. It took seeing her friend's success to make her realize that she too was employable. If June had tried brainstorming, she might have written down a number of jobs that she felt capable of doing. Having written them down, she might then have tried finding out what sort of qualifications and experience applicants were expected to have. While making these enquiries, she might then have been surprised to learn that the local play-centre would be willing to employ her.

Brainstorming will help you to get out of the habit of saying 'Yes, but . . .' Remember, there is plenty of time available in which to evaluate your ideas. So, suspend your judgement and let the ideas come thick and fast!

Making decisions

Weighing up the pros and cons

The next stage of problem-solving is deciding what to do. A good way to start doing this is to list the pros and cons associated with each answer to your problem. Pros are the good things associated with a particular decision, and cons are the bad things or drawbacks. As always, the best way to explain this is by using an example.

Sue

Sue is worried about her job prospects. She has been working as a laboratory technician in a hospital for the past five years. However, she is bored with her job and has begun worrying about her future. She has started to get thoughts like 'What am I doing with my life? I can't be enthusiastic about my work any more. If I carry on like this, then I'm going to be trapped in a job that I'm not enjoying.'

Sue has finished brainstorming. She thought up six ways of dealing with the problem. However, in order to make this explanation clearer, we will only look at two of her possible solutions. Her first solution was a complete career change. Sue had once been a voluntary counsellor at an advice centre and had enjoyed it very much. So she found the idea of becoming a professional counsellor very appealing. Her second solution was to try to make her job as a laboratory technician more interesting. She considered this possible by taking a more active role in her department.

So, what are the pros and cons associated with these two solutions? Table 3.1 shows the sort of lists that Sue might make.

We can see that there are more pros than cons associated with becoming a counsellor, whereas there are more cons than pros

Table 3.1 Sue's solutions

Solution one: Career change?

Pros	Cons
I'll really enjoy being a counsellor.	I'll have to get a new qualification.
I might be able to work from home: no long journeys on the train!	If I become self-employed, this will be risky. What if nobody comes to see me?
I wouldn't be stuck in front of the computer any more. I always find that difficult.	If I have to study again, I'll have to do a part-time course. This will damage my social life.
When I'm qualified I might have more free time.	

Solution two: Taking a more active role?

Pros	Cons
I might get a pay rise.	I'll have to be more forceful. This is quite difficult in my department.
My life won't be disrupted.	I'll have to work a lot harder.
	I may be asked to give talks on special topics. I hate talking in public.
	I'll have to see a lot more of the head of the department. We never get on very well.

associated with taking a more active role at work. It would seem, then, that Sue would be better off changing her job.

However, just counting up pros and cons can be misleading. All pros are not equally advantageous, and not all cons are equally problematic. For example, let us imagine an individual who is evaluating the merits of two jobs. In the pros column of the first job the following is written: 'I will double my income.' However, in the pros column of the second job we find: 'I will be able to have an extra five-minute tea break.' Clearly, the pro relating to the first job (doubled income) is considerably more important than the pro relating to the second job (additional tea break).

A way of getting around this problem is by placing a number, called a weighting, next to each pro and each con. The weighting represents how important each statement is. It's usually a good idea to do this by picking a number between 1 and 10. There is a slight limitation here, in that your most important item cannot be rated as more than ten times as important as your least important item. Because of this, some people find it easier to rate items using a wider range, say between 1 and 50. However, there are no hard and fast rules: choose a scale that you feel comfortable with. Table 3.2 shows what Sue's lists will look like with weightings included.

Bear in mind that Table 3.2 is a very crude example of a list of pros and cons. When making a serious career decision, it is not always possible to reduce the advantages and disadvantages in this way. A pros and cons list is a way of helping you to decide which potential solution to choose. A number of books give the impression that this technique is a powerful method of assisting decision-making, but perhaps this is over-optimistic. A more sensible view is that making a list of good and bad consequences helps you to clarify issues associated with a particular decision. In other words, putting things down on paper might help you to make vague feelings more concrete. Also, assigning values to particular statements might prompt you to think about the consequences more thoroughly.

A minor problem with this technique is that after adding up the pros and cons associated with two options, the numbers you get at the end may be about the same. This means that you still have to choose the better option. However, having looked at the issues more closely, such a decision might be a little easier. Also, if you know that both options are favourable, then you don't stand to lose much either way.

Some people find that after adding up the pros and cons the numbers tell them that a first solution is better than a second solution. However, they still feel reluctant to go ahead with their first solution. There are a number of ways of looking at such an outcome. Sometimes, we just don't feel right about a particular decision, even when the evidence is in favour of it. Under these circumstances it's a good idea to talk things over with someone

Table 3.2 Sue's scores

Solution one: Career change?

Pros		Cons	
I'll really enjoy being a counsellor.	8	I'll have to get a new qualification.	3
I might be able to work from home: no long journeys on the train!	5	If I become self-employed, this will be risky. What if nobody comes to see me?	7
I wouldn't be stuck in front of the computer any more. I always find that difficult.	3	If I have to study again, I'll have to do a part-time course. This will damage my social life.	5
When I'm qualified I might have more free time.	7		
TOTAL	**23**		**15**

If we add up the weightings we find that the total for pros is 23, whereas the total for cons is 15. The difference between 23 and 15 is 8, in favour of pros. In other words, there are more good things associated with becoming a counsellor than bad things.

Solution two: Taking a more active role?

Pros		Cons	
I might get a pay rise.	4	I'll have to be more forceful. This is quite difficult in my department.	7
My life won't be disrupted.	7	I'll have to work a lot harder.	6
		I may be asked to give talks on special topics. I hate talking in public.	5
		I'll have to see a lot more of the head of the department. We never get on very well.	7
TOTAL	**11**		**25**

The difference between 11 and 25 is 14, in favour of cons. This means that there are more drawbacks associated with trying to take a more active role in the department than there are good things. Clearly, the best decision for Sue is to change career. This appears to be the best plan.

in order to get to the bottom of those reservations. Perhaps your lists are incomplete, in that there are some things that need to be written down that you've missed out. On the other hand, perhaps the problem is so complex that it just cannot be reduced to a list of 'for' and 'against' items. Remember, listing pros and cons is simply a helpful way of clarifying issues. Feeling uncomfortable about the outcome of a particular set of pros and cons might be a necessary step towards uncovering a deeper problem. Let's take another example.

Alice

Alice was offered two jobs. The first was a well-paid management position in a large department store fairly close to her home. The second wasn't so well paid, and involved working as a secretary in the office of an interior design company. After doing a pros and cons analysis she wasn't surprised to find that there were many more advantages associated with taking up the management job. However, she just didn't feel right. Although there would be more money, more responsibility and good promotion prospects if she took the management job, she just didn't want to do it. After considering the situation, she came to the following conclusions. She had never really enjoyed working in management. The only reason that she had taken management posts in the past was to secure a good income. Because her husband and family had always encouraged her to apply for well-paid jobs, she had got into a 'management rut'. Now that she had a choice, she could see that 'money' wasn't really her priority. She had always been interested in design, and would have perhaps gone to a design college had her parents not 'bullied' her into taking business studies. Her pros and cons analysis reflected more of what her husband and family wanted her to do than what she wanted to do herself. Her real inclination was to take the secretarial post, so that she could see how a design company worked. Although she hadn't admitted it to herself for a long time, she still wanted to study design. Therefore, she was attracted to a working environment where she could watch designers doing their job on a day-to-day basis.

When choosing between options, you have to ask yourself not only 'What do I want?' but also 'What do I *really* want?'. This is because our *real* needs aren't always easy to recognize. Some psychologists and counsellors ask their clients to make a distinction between *self* and *self-concept*. The *self* is 'you', who you really are. The *self-concept* is the 'you' that owes much to the expectations and values of others. As we develop as people, we often accept ideas and values that have very little to do with us. When we make decisions, we may feel uncomfortable because the decision has been influenced by our *self*-concept, more than our true *self*.

When you make a decision, ask: 'Why do I want to do this?' Is it because you want to do it? Or is it because you think it is the correct and proper thing to do? If so, correct and proper by whose standards? Yours? Or your parents'? If you have a voice in your head saying that you 'should' solve your problem this way, or that you 'ought to' solve your problem that way, then question it!

There is in fact very little in this life that you 'should' or 'ought to' do. Statements worded in this way are probably closer to your parents' or somebody else's wishes rather than yours. If you use a pros and cons analysis and are still feeling unsure, then reconsider how you weighted the pros and cons. Do the values reflect your feelings, or someone else's?

If we become sensitive to our true feelings, then this might have a dramatic effect on how we view decisions. We might choose to give up striving to achieve something, because when we look at the achievement we see it has more to do with other people's wishes than our own. Giving up, under these circumstances, is a successful decision. In our example above, Alice recognizes that she wants to give up the chance of a well-paid job in management. However, this decision is a successful decision in her terms. Although her husband and family might not think so, to Alive the decision to 'give up' on management is the correct decision. It feels right. The closer your decisions are to your own wishes, rather than other people's, the more comfortable you will be with them. This is not only true of 'giving up' decisions, it is also true of 'go-for-it' decisions. Recognizing what you want for yourself might have the effect of inspiring you to consider choices that you previously failed to acknowledge. Perhaps your parents and other significant people in your life have always discouraged you from taking certain types of decision.

Earlier, we said that a pros and cons analysis might not work because the lists were incomplete. However, it might be the case that there is sufficient evidence available for you to make a decision but you still can't choose. This is a major problem for worriers! You will recall that in Chapter 1 it was suggested that worriers are generally slower than non-worriers when making decisions. In the next section we will consider this very important point in more detail.

Learning to make quicker decisions

We said in Chapter 1 that worry fills the time between realizing that something is wrong and doing something about it. So, the longer you take to decide on a course of action, the longer you will worry and suffer the consequences. So, swifter decision-making is likely to reduce the amount of time you spend worrying.

Now, if you are an inveterate worrier, you are likely to have some fairly strong beliefs about quick decisions. You will probably be naturally cautious, and feel that a quick decision means taking unnecessary risks. This sort of thinking is epitomized in proverbs such as 'More haste, less speed'. This proverb is actually a very old one; even the ancient Romans had an equivalent saying – 'Festina lente', which means 'Hasten slowly.' The fact is that this proverb, like all proverbs, tells the truth, but not the whole truth! Of course making hasty decisions and rushing into things is a bad idea. However, this doesn't mean that making a quick decision is always wrong. Further, if you have defined your problem carefully and considered the pros and cons associated with several ways of coping, you can hardly be accused of rushing into something.

In Chapter 1 we considered briefly the mechanisms that delay decision-making in worriers. We said that worriers often demand more evidence than is readily available, in an attempt to be absolutely sure that they are doing the right thing. The word 'evidence' is used here to mean information relevant to a particular decision. When you are choosing between coping strategies, it is necessary at some point to accept the evidence favouring the selection of one above the others. If you do not accept such evidence, you will be paralysed by indecision. You will find yourself going over the same things again and again, in an effort to be absolutely sure that what you are about to do is correct.

Life would be considerably easier if we could predict the future. The popularity of astrology columns in magazines and newspapers gives us some idea of how powerful this 'need to know' actually is. Even the most rational people will sometimes have a quick look at their 'stars'. Astrology has remained popular because, for many people, living with uncertainty is quite difficult. Astrology can be comforting, in that it appears to take away some of that uncertainty.

Unfortunately, it really is impossible to know the future, whatever we might want to believe. When we select a coping strategy, we are simply choosing to do something that, to the best of our knowledge, has a good chance of achieving a desired goal. All decisions are risky decisions in that sense. There is no such thing as a decision that has no risk attached to it. Going down the road to buy a loaf of bread could be seen as a highly risky business: you might get run over! The baker might decide to shoot you! An aeroplane might crash on your head! It is always possible to think of things that can go wrong. These examples are admittedly bizarre; however, worriers can delay decision-making because of this kind of thinking. A worrier who has defined a problem might know exactly what options are available, but feel that there isn't enough evidence favouring one in particular.

So, how do we go about making quicker decisions? The first thing you can do is become accustomed to taking *sensible risks*. Although we cannot know with absolute certainty what is going to happen, we all have enough life experience to have a pretty good guess. For our purposes, exact knowledge is unnecessary. Start by making quicker decisions about things where the consequences are not too serious either way.

You needn't wait for a problem to do this. You can make quicker decisions about choosing between pleasant options. For example, you might be in a bookshop with a small amount of money, having noticed two books you really like. Do a quick pros and cons analysis of each in your head, then just go ahead and buy one. Don't stand there for ages thinking about how you might make the wrong decision. You can't possibly know which book will be more enjoyable yet, because you haven't read either. All that you can say at this point is that you seem to like both of them. In addition, it isn't really that important to know which is the absolute best. If the purpose of going to a bookshop is to buy a book, then that is easily accomplished! Remember, even if the book you buy turns out to be less enjoyable than you thought, does it really matter? Worriers have a habit of turning minor problems into major catastrophes. You can always buy the other book some other time!

The above example is interesting in that it shows how worriers can find something to worry about in the least threatening situations. There is nothing inherently 'threatening' in the act of choosing a book. However, the worrier will be able to make the situation unpleasant by thinking about failing to make the best possible choice, instead of thinking: 'I'll enjoy both of them to some extent, whichever one I buy, so I may as well buy this one.'

After you have practised making simple decisions more swiftly, have a go at harder ones. You might give yourself a deadline. If the deadline arrives and you're still unsure, make your decision anyway. If you are used to being very cautious, then 'jumping in at the deep end' will feel quite unpleasant at first. However, with practice you will learn that resolving your problems faster means you have less to worry about. Feeling a little uncomfortable after making a quick decision is a small price to pay for worry reduction. Also, this discomfort is likely to pass. As you learn that faster decision-making isn't always followed by a major catastrophe, you will find it easier and easier to do. Perhaps you should write down your decisions, the time it took you to make them, and then what happened as a result. A written record will remind you that taking sensible risks results in *less* worry, not *more* disasters.

So what are the key points to remember?

- Worry will fill up the time between recognizing a 'threat' or problem, and dealing with it.
- The quicker you deal with your problem, the less time you will spend worrying.
- There is never enough evidence available to ensure that your decision is absolutely right; there are always risks.
- If you have defined your problem carefully and evaluated ways of coping with that problem, you are not being rash or hasty.
- Finally, if you have begun to act on the basis of one of your decisions, see it through. All decisions have pros and cons. Don't focus on the cons! It is easy to regret making a decision if you only think about associated drawbacks. Always remind yourself of the advantages!

Being realistic

When the idea of brainstorming was introduced, you were asked to suspend judgement. This was suggested to encourage you to think up as many solutions as possible, and to discourage a tendency to say 'Yes, but . . .' However, once you have generated a number of coping strategies, it is important to be realistic. Don't attempt to solve a problem in a way that might be beyond your capabilities. Although it isn't a good idea to limit yourself, neither is it a good idea to attempt to solve a problem in a way to which you are not suited. We all have limitations. Sometimes, our circumstances make us test those limitations, but this can lead to disappointment or pleasant surprise. Clearly it depends on how difficult the task is, and how suited we are to coping with it. Let's take another example.

Fred
At the age of 52 Fred was unlucky enough to have a heart attack. This made him stop and seriously reconsider his lifestyle. His diet was atrocious, and he spent every working day behind a desk. Fred's idea of exercise was walking to the car so that he could drive to work. Fred's doctor told him to start eating a healthy diet, and to make the effort to engage in some sort of activity on a regular basis. Unfortunately, Fred decided to start jogging. He had never jogged before, and soon found it impossible to maintain a regular exercise routine. His legs began to ache, and he ended up skipping most of his so-called 'activity sessions'. His doctor told him that he was trying to do too much, too soon, and suggested he try swimming instead. Fred found swimming a great deal easier, and was able to keep up a pattern of regular exercise. The point here is to try to avoid disappointment by selecting strategies with which you have a sporting chance of succeeding.

For some people, failure becomes habitual. Indeed, setting unrealistic goals and constantly failing can be reassuring. If you know that you are going to fail, the world is less unpredictable. Perhaps more importantly, if you know that you are going to fail, you can avoid all the effort involved in dealing with a troublesome situation. Some people use their own 'incompetence' and 'helplessness' as a manipulative tool. The underlying assumption is: 'If I can't do it, then somebody else will have to do it for me.' Sadly, not all of our problems can be shifted onto the shoulders of others. So, do be careful. If you find that you are attracted to ways of solving problems that have never proved effective for you in the past, then think again. Try to select a coping strategy that you might have used successfully before. If you can't think of one, then make a list of things that you're good at. Would any of these skills be useful when attempting to solve your problem? Do they correspond with the demands of the coping strategy you have selected?

If you don't have much self-confidence, then you probably don't think you have many skills to fall back on. You might, for example, think that you're not very clever. However, being 'clever' isn't all that important. You might be a very 'warm' person. As it happens, being 'warm' is a 'skill' that a lot of so-called clever people haven't acquired! Being 'warm' might be a really important characteristic for the success of a particular coping strategy. So, don't adopt a narrow view of what constitutes a skill. You probably have a wealth of skills, but as yet don't regard them as such.

To summarize then, when attempting to select a solution to your problem, first use a pros and cons analysis to clarify issues and sort out which strategy will give you the best possible outcome. Second, consider how well equipped you are. By all means take up a difficult challenge, but by the same token don't attempt to solve a problem that demands skills you do not have, or are unlikely to acquire.

Implementing your coping strategy

The next stage in problem-solving is to actually implement your coping strategy. In other words, you now have to act on your decision. We have already noted that worriers tend to be reluctant to make decisions and act on them. So, remind yourself that unless you solve your problem, you will keep on experiencing worry. The whole point of using problem-solving is to work out a successful way of dealing with whatever it is that's causing you to worry in the first place. Turn your worry into actions as soon as possible.

Evaluation

The final stage in problem-solving is evaluating your progress. Did the coping strategy you selected deal with the problem? If the answer is yes, then well done. It's always a good idea to give yourself a pat on the back when you have achieved something, or an immediate treat. If you are not used to treating yourself, then make a reward menu. Make a list of things that you like, such as going to the cinema or buying some new clothes. When you have successfully resolved a problem, indulge yourself! Rewards don't have to be big. A book or magazine might be sufficient. The main thing is to acknowledge your own success.

Rewards work by *reinforcing* behaviours. When psychologists say that something is 'reinforcing', they mean that it will increase the chances of that behaviour occurring again. This simple principle is one that has been frequently tested by psychologists, and found to be true. It doesn't only work for humans, it also works for animals. In fact, 'reinforcement schedules' were originally developed by a psychologist called B. F. Skinner, using rats and pigeons in a laboratory! If your successes are rewarded, then you will be more likely to repeat whatever you did to accomplish those successes. So, if you reward your successful problem-solving, you will be more likely to engage in 'problem-solving' the next time you have a problem.

If your coping strategy has failed, so what? It really isn't the end of the world. You can always have another go. Go back to your list of alternative ways of dealing with the problem – that is, the list compiled after brainstorming – and select another strategy. If this doesn't seem right, then you can always go right back to the beginning, the problem definition stage, and redefine your problem. As we said earlier, it is easy to confuse problems.

Also, remember that some things look easier to do 'on paper' than they are in real life. For example, there has been much written on being assertive. This is often presented as the answer to a number of problems, which indeed it can be. However, it is easy to confuse knowing about assertiveness with actually *being* assertive. If you are a shy person, then being assertive takes a lot of practice. Just knowing about it isn't enough. Knowing when and how to be assertive are skills that take some time to acquire.

The above is not written to discourage you from attending assertiveness training groups. As already stated, assertiveness just might be the answer to some of your problems. However, the point here is that if assertiveness training is right for you, then you will need to practise being assertive to get the benefit of the training. Knowing about it doesn't automatically make you assertive.

As we said earlier, problem-solving is a skill. Knowing about the principles is not enough. You have to practise putting those principles into action. You may find that before you can deal with worrying problems, you need a great deal of practice. Don't be discouraged by setbacks. Don't fall into the trap of thinking that one setback means that you will always fail. Although setbacks are upsetting, don't allow them to put you off having another go. We have already stressed that it is impossible to know the future. Treat each new attempt to solve your problem as if it is the first.

A final consideration:
will problem-solving really stop me worrying?

Before closing this chapter it is worthwhile considering a very important question: 'Will problem-solving work for me?' Although it is impossible to guarantee success, there is enough evidence to suggest that applying the techniques outlined in this chapter will help you to deal with the problems more effectively. If you are dealing with your problems more effectively, then you should have less to worry about.

A few years ago a treatment package was developed in the USA for people described as 'chronic worriers'. These were people who reported worrying for 50 per cent of the day or more. They were basically given the following instructions.

• Learn to identify worrisome thoughts and other thoughts that are unnecessary or unpleasant; distinguish these from necessary or pleasant thoughts related to the present moment.
• Establish a half-hour worry period to take place at the same time and in the same location each day.

- When you catch yourself worrying, postpone the worry to the worry period and replace it with attending to present-moment experience.
- Make use of the half-hour worry period to worry about your concerns and to engage in problem-solving to eliminate those worries.

At the end of the study, those people who had been treated reported that they worried much less than before. These instructions have much in common with the suggestions included in this chapter. They stress learning to recognize worry and the importance of problem-solving. The only real difference is the suggestion that worry should be ignored until a half-hour worry period. The ability to dismiss worries is something that not everybody has. Therefore, it may be better for some people to deal with worry at the earliest opportunity.

However, you might be good at stopping yourself worrying, in which case these particular instructions may be of some use. As we said earlier, worry is largely uninvited. We tend to worry at times when it is not possible to sit down quietly in order to define our problems. If you find that you worry a lot when, for example, you are at work or busy looking after children, then perhaps practising postponement is something you should try.

It might be an idea to remind yourself at this point how postponement might be achieved. If you recall, earlier we discussed distraction and 'distancing yourself' from the worry process. By distraction, we mean trying to occupy the mind with something else other than worry – going shopping or reading a good book. Distancing yourself from worry means not getting drawn into thinking about the distressing thoughts and images that start you worrying. In other words, you try to act the way you do when the television is on but you're not really watching it. You are aware of the images on the screen, but you don't get involved with the 'story'. In the same way, you can be aware of 'worry' images entering your head, but at the same time refuse to think about them. With practice, it might be possible for you to develop the ability to shut out worry more effectively. If you can do this, postponing your worries until a half-hour worry period each day might be useful.

4

Problem-solving in action

In Chapter 3 we described a problem-solving package. However, you should note that it isn't the only way to go about solving your problems. As we said earlier, a problem-solving package is simply a set of suggestions or instructions that might be useful when dealing with a common problem. You may find that it's possible to modify this approach so that it is particularly useful for you. For example, you might find thinking about your problems easier when prompted with questions. You might therefore choose to make a list of questions which reflect the stages of problem-solving presented in Chapter 3. These might be written down as in Table 4.1.

Table 4.1 Problem-solving stages

- What am I worried about?
- What do I want to happen?
- What can I do to make it happen?
- What is actually likely to happen?
- What is my decision?

And after you have implemented your coping strategy:

- Did it work?

Here's an example of how these questions can prompt useful answers.

Anna

Put yourself in the position of Anna. She is 20, and lives on her own in an area where mugging is an all too frequent occurrence.

Although Anna was well aware that this sort of thing went on, she wasn't unduly concerned about it. However, in a short space of time, two of her friends were 'bothered' for money while coming home late at night. Neither were hurt, but both were upset by the experience. Since talking to them, Anna has started to worry. She asks herself the following questions:

- *What am I worried about?*
  I don't seem to go out as much as I used too. I'm worried that I'll get out of touch with my friends. I used to go out every Friday and Saturday, but now I only go out about once every three weeks. Why? Well, it's not that I don't enjoy going out. I think it's because I'm reluctant to go out. Coming back late could be dangerous. So, I'm really worried about getting mugged when I come home late.
- *What do I want to happen?*
  I want to be able to go out, enjoy myself and come back as late as I like without having to worry about the possibility of being mugged.
- *What can I do to make it happen?*
  I could learn to drive. I could learn self-defence. I could share a cab with my friends. I could always go home with a friend: she could stay over at my place, or vice versa.
- *What is actually likely to happen?*
  Although I might learn to drive one day, I don't really have the money for lessons at present, and I certainly couldn't afford a car. Self-defence is a good idea, but I can't see myself going to classes every week; I'm not very good at seeing things through. Sharing a cab with a friend would be possible – but I'd have to remember to put some money aside each week, and find out who is willing to share before arranging anything. Staying over is reasonable, although that might not always be convenient.
- *What is my decision?*
  I think I'll put money aside for a cab, and make sure that there's somebody who is willing to share.
- *Did it work?*
  Yes. I went out on Saturday. I got a cab in the West End with Kirsty. It didn't work out too expensive and I was dropped

off just outside my front door. The driver waited for me to get inside before he drove off. I will do this again next week.

There is nothing 'sacred' about the approach described in Chapter 3, and you can 'tamper' with each stage if you wish. The only thing you shouldn't change is the order. Clearly, you cannot do something about a problem before you have defined it! The great advantage of problem-solving approaches is that they allow you to break problems down in a systematic way. It is much easier to deal with a problem in small steps that follow on logically from each other than to deal with a problem in one go. Everyday problems can often feel as though they are about to get 'out of control'. Problem-solving is a way you can regain control over your life and re-establish some sort of order.

Another thing to remember is that you might be quite good at some aspects of problem-solving already, in which case you may find some of the steps outlined in Chapter 3 more useful than others. As we have already stressed, most worriers find decision-making particularly difficult. If you recognize that you have trouble 'making your mind up', then it would be better to devote more time to practising this skill compared with, say, problem definition. You may find defining your problems and generating coping strategies quite easy. Remember, a problem-solving package is only a rough guide. You can be flexible in your approach, making greater use of the hints and directions that you find particularly helpful.

Problem-solving examples

In this chapter we are going to look at how the problem-solving package described in Chapter 3 works in real life. Although examples have been given before, these have not been detailed examples, showing you how the package might work from start to finish. We will take three characters, Jo, Andrew and Jane. All are experiencing worry because of a current problem.

Jo

Jo was beginning to feel uneasy. She had started to feel tense, and found concentrating on her work difficult. At first she ignored these feelings, but then one day she sat down and decided to work out what was going on. Christmas had come and gone, leaving her with an outstanding credit card debt, on top of a number of bills from the previous year that had to be paid. However, she knew that this happened every January. Financial problems had never made her feel this uneasy. She always managed to work her way out of debt in the end.

Jo then started to think about her relationship with David. Jo and David had been living together for six months. Before living together, they had been a couple for about a year. Jo's mother had disapproved of them living together, and this had caused some family arguments. Jo had said at the time that they were very much in love, and that she 'knew what she was doing'. Because Jo had been so adamant that her relationship with David was working, she was now reluctant to admit to herself that things weren't going very well. In spite of this natural reluctance, Jo recognized that for several months she had been 'worrying' about the future. Instead of considering these worries carefully she had ignored them in the hope that they would just 'go away' and things would 'work out'. Jo had been able to ignore these worries quite successfully. During the day she was able to throw herself wholeheartedly into her work. However, at night she was more vulnerable. In the moments before sleep, with her defences down, these thoughts were more difficult to block out. She had attributed their frequent occurrence to tiredness. She had also convinced herself that if she took these worries too seriously she would be 'making a mountain out of a molehill'. Now, Jo recognized that these worries were acting like an alarm system, telling her that something was wrong and needed to be dealt with.

Once Jo had acknowledged that something was wrong, she was ready to start problem-solving. Her first step was to define the problem more accurately. She recognized that her relationship was somehow different, but she wasn't sure in what way it was different. David wasn't being unkind in any way, and she still enjoyed being with him. However, Jo began to think about their life on a day-to-day basis, and realized that they weren't spending as much time together as they used to. In fact, she was now seeing less of David than ever before. They seemed to be growing apart.

Their relationship had lost some of its intimacy, and Jo missed the closeness they once shared. David was not a very communicative person, and Jo doubted whether she could get him to talk about it. Why was he going out so much? Jo suspected that living together had made David think about marriage. Although Jo had expressed no desire to get married, she felt that David had come to see their life together as a commitment in that direction. It was possible that he now regretted 'moving in', but was unable to express his regret. People who find it difficult to put things into words often express their feelings by behaving differently – and David was certainly behaving differently. Jo realized that if nothing was done soon, they might drift so far apart that the stability of their relationship would be under threat. She had begun to worry about what sort of a future she might have without David. She had also begun to imagine sitting in front of her mother and announcing that the relationship was over. In her imagination, Jo could clearly hear her mother saying, 'I told you living together was a bad idea!'

Jo then began to think of ways she might cope with the situation. After brainstorming, she wrote down the following situations:

- Go back to living separately again while maintaining a commitment to each other. This might make the relationship work again.
- Live apart without a commitment to each other for a few months. This might stop David feeling trapped. It would also give me a chance to see what life is like without David.
- Ask David to go with me to see a counsellor.
- Have an affair, to see if I can get the closeness elsewhere that our relationship lacks.
- Finish the relationship and start another one. If we can't live together now, then maybe it just isn't going to work ever.

At first Jo thought that living apart again while maintaining a commitment would be the best solution. However, there were some significant disadvantages associated with this choice. She would still have to face her mother, and it felt to Jo like 'a step backwards'. Jo thought that asking David to see a counsellor was one of her less realistic options. He was reluctant to talk to her, so she felt it unlikely that he would 'bare his soul' to a stranger. However, she reconsidered this point. Perhaps a counsellor would be skilled enough to get David talking. If that were possible, then perhaps it would be better in the long run.

After doing a pros and cons analysis of all her choices, she decided that seeking help might be the best thing to do. There was a big drawback associated with this decision. David might simply say 'No', then it would be a complete non-starter. However, Jo recognized that all her choices had risks associated with them, and if nothing was done the relationship would probably end anyway. It was best to make a decision and get it over with.

When Jo asked David if he would see a counsellor, she was surprised to hear him agree. He was aware that he had been behaving differently, and felt a little confused. He felt that talking his feelings over with somebody else around would be less intense, and was likely to be more productive. The following day Jo implemented the strategy by making an arrangement to see a counsellor who specialized in relationship problems.

A month later Jo evaluated her strategy. She and David were getting on much better than before, although going to see a counsellor had brought to light a lot of things concerning their relationship that were unexpected. Nevertheless, overall their relationship had improved, and they seemed to be happier together.

The above example shows how important it is not to predict the future. Jo had assumed at first that because David had trouble talking about his feelings to her, he would also have trouble talking to somebody else. In fact, David saw the situation very differently. By brainstorming, Jo forced herself to evaluate an idea which could have easily been dismissed. A second point here is that if a problem is complicated, it's all right to seek outside help. This help might be consulting someone who has access to information relating to one of your problems, or someone who can help in a more involved way, like a counsellor. If you make a decision to seek help, that's a perfectly legitimate way of dealing with your problem. Although it might be argued that Jo didn't solve the problem directly, she used the process of problem-solving to get her one step nearer to a solution. You may find that problem-solving doesn't always solve your problems, but allows you to get closer to a solution each time you use it.

Andrew

Andrew had been invited to a dinner party, a large gathering, with a group of about ten guests. Even as he wrote the date in his diary he began to feel apprehensive. By the time the engagement was less than a fortnight away, Andrew had begun to worry about it. All of a sudden he would remember the dinner party and feel 'uneasy'. He imagined himself sitting at the dinner table, saying stupid things. He also imagined how people might talk about him unfavourably after he had left.

Andrew decided it was time to get to the bottom of his worries, so he sat down with a pencil and paper, ready to define the problem. He realized that in the past he had always found dinner parties difficult to cope with. There were a number of things that seemed to be expected of him that he didn't really like doing. For instance, he didn't like dressing up. Being smart always made him feel self-conscious. However, more important than this was the fact that he found 'small talk' quite difficult. He could never think of anything to say during dinner.

Andrew quite enjoyed talking to people one at a time. He was also quite capable of sustaining an interesting conversation in a small group. Andrew had a number of interests, and more often than not he would meet someone who shared some of these interests after dinner. However, the dinner itself was always a problem. He always felt stupid and unable to contribute anything to the conversation. Also, talking to a large group of people made him nervous. He always felt as though he were making some kind of public speech!

Andrew saw that he felt stupid largely because he had nothing to say. He then asked himself why that was the case. He tried to remember how things usually went for the first hour or so at most parties. During dinner, people tended to talk about things he knew nothing about. He wasn't particularly interested in current affairs, and didn't watch much television. However, these seemed to be the main topics of conversation during dinner. When somebody asked him what he though of 'this' or 'that' item of news, he always felt incredibly stupid being forced to admit that he knew nothing about it. Andrew realized that the main reason why he had nothing to say was quite straightforward. He really didn't have anything to say!

Andrew considered how he might cope with the situation. After brainstorming he wrote down the following solutions:

- I don't have to go, I can always cancel.
- I don't have to go to the dinner, I can ring up the host the day before and say I will be arriving late.
- I can always get drunk, then nobody will expect me to say anything sensible.
- I can read the newspapers and watch the news regularly before I go; this way I might be able to join in the conversation more easily.

Andrew wasn't always good at making decisions, For a few days he found it difficult to decide whether he really wanted to go to the party at all. He found himself saying 'Shall I, shan't I?' Andrew saw that this indecisive state was feeding his worry, so he made a firm decision that he would definitely go to the party, and resolved to choose an appropriate coping strategy by the following evening.

At first, Andrew thought that ringing the host the day before and saying he would be unavoidably delayed was quite a good idea. But then, he thought about how this would mean 'walking in' on a group of people who had already been together for most of the evening. This would make him feel an 'outsider' from the moment he arrived. After a pros and cons analysis of his 'coping strategies' he decided that reading the newspapers and watching the news would be sufficient for him to deal with dinner party small talk. Andrew had never prepared for a party before, and appreciated that if this strategy was successful, he might continue to 'define' and 'deal with' other problems of a similar nature. Clearly, this would be of enormous long-term benefit.

Andrew went to the party and had an enjoyable evening. He was able to join in with the small talk, and after dinner felt that he knew people well enough to talk about the sort of things he felt more comfortable discussing. He got on very well with someone called Mary, who invited him over to her place for dinner the following week. When Andrew evaluated his strategy, he considered it very successful!

Andrew saw the next dinner party he was invited to as another opportunity for coping. As you will remember, dressing up made him feel self-conscious, so two days before the next party he took to wearing his dinner jacket around the house. By the time he went to the party, he had got so used to wearing it that putting it on had no effect on him whatsoever! Needless to say, he had also studied the papers and watched the news very carefully.

Like Andrew, you might have a problem which can be broken down into a number of parts. If you are worried about entering a particular situation, then deal with a new part every time you enter it. In our example, Andrew dealt with the most difficult part first. For him, this was making conversation over dinner. After coping with this problem, he went on to cope with the less stressful difficulty of feeling uncomfortable when dressed up. However, you don't have to tackle your most demanding problems first. You might find it easier to work up to big problems by attempting to cope with smaller ones first.

Jane

Jane worked in a computer employment agency, where occasionally she was asked to prepare staff reports and present appropriate facts and figures. Her presentation was required in a week's time. Unfortunately she had prepared a presentation that she knew was below her usual standard. Jane had recently started dating a new boyfriend; consequently, she had been going out more than usual. The time that she would usually spend staying late at work – getting things 'just right' – had been spent going out and having fun.

Jane did not find it difficult defining the problem. She was worried that she would be asked questions that she could not answer by the company directors. These meetings were quite important. Promotion often depended on consistent high-quality presentations. Jane knew that her last presentation but one could have been better. At the time it didn't seem to matter, because she was usually very diligent at work. However, at that time she had not anticipated a new relationship and all the distractions of the past month. So, in summary, Jane was not happy with her presentation, and was expecting a long meeting punctuated by difficult questions which she would be unable to answer.

Jane considered her alternatives:

- I can rework my presentation entirely.
- I can rework the weakest parts of the presentation only.
- I can pretend that I'm ill, and cancel the meeting.
- I can ask one of the directors for more time.
- I can present my report as it is, and hope that nobody notices that it is below standard.

At first, Jane quite liked the idea of going off sick. However, this would mean cancelling other engagements that she really needed to attend. Reworking her presentation entirely meant late nights at work for the next week. She knew that not only would this be very tiring, affecting her work performance during the day, it would also interfere with her social life. She finally decided that the best thing to do would be to accept a compromise solution. She would put in a few late nights attempting to salvage the weakest parts of her report. This, she felt, would be reasonable. After all, if the work wasn't too patchy, the directors might not even notice.

Jane was able to spend the next three evenings working late. This wasn't too disruptive, and she felt adequately prepared. The rest of the week she was able to spend enjoying herself, free of worry and confident that the presentation would be of a sufficient standard.

5

Coping with setbacks

If you have read the last few chapters carefully, then you should be fairly well acquainted by now with the techniques associated with problem-solving. You will know that worry can be used to identify problem areas in your life, and that the appropriate response to worry is systematic problem-solving. For most people, worry leads to more worry, instead of decisions and actions. In order to worry less, you must learn to replace worry with problem-solving at the earliest opportunity. In the past, perhaps worry has always signalled a sleepless night or a headache. These associations must be broken. When you worry now, you must think of worry as a cue, a signal that tells you a problem needs defining. If worry is always followed by problem-solving, then a strong association will develop.

Hopefully, after sufficient practice, problem-solving will become automatic. Worry will stop being followed by more worry, and start to be followed by the first stage of problem-solving without much mental effort. Over several months, the association that exists between worry and tension will be broken, and replaced with the far more useful association between worry and problem-solving. In other words, you will have 'kicked' a bad habit, and replaced it with a good one. But to get to the point where problem-solving becomes an automatic response will require practice. You might remember that practice was stressed in Chapter 2. So, practise problem-solving whenever you can. Treat even your trivial worries as an opportunity to engage in problem-solving.

Sadly, things don't always go the way you want them to. Although you might be quite successful resolving most of your problems, it is unlikely that you will be successful resolving all of them. You are bound to make a few mistakes. You might define a problem incorrectly. You might choose the wrong coping strategy.

You might even attempt to solve a problem that simply *cannot* be solved. If you are the sort of person who feels disappointments keenly, then this chapter is especially for you. In it, we are going to consider how we might protect ourselves from 'giving up' because of 'failures'.

You have no doubt heard of inoculation, where the body produces antibodies to attack specific germs. This chapter is a way of inoculating yourself psychologically against 'failures'. Instead of building up antibodies, we are going to build up a store of coping thoughts. These will combat the negative thoughts that tempt us to 'give up', in the same way that real antibodies combat germs. Now that you know about problem-solving, it would be unfortunate if a few setbacks stopped you from practising it. Before we consider psychological inoculation, we must provide some background information.

Thoughts and feelings: a close relationship

We will start off by taking a look at thoughts and feelings. Hopefully, by the end of this chapter you will see that how you feel has a lot to do with what you are thinking. We will then take a look at negative thinking, and consider how bad thoughts can make us feel bad. These bad feelings often cause us to take a pessimistic view of our own ability to cope with problems. Finally, we will consider the kind of thoughts that are likely to make us 'give up' trying to cope with our problems. We will learn to identify these thoughts, and then we will learn how to make them less harmful. This process is similar to bomb disposal. After we have found our most destructive thoughts, we then set about disarming them!

In everyday speech we often discriminate between thoughts and feelings. We treat them as though they have nothing to do with each other. This view is typical of certain stereotypes that appear in fiction and on television. People who think a lot, for example scientists, are often depicted as calculating, logical, cold and uninspired. They work in laboratories, where they spend more time with computers than with other people. On the other hand, people who feel things deeply, for example artists, are depicted as spontaneous, intuitive, warm and creative. These stereotypes couldn't be further from the truth. Scientists often work on 'hunches', and make their discoveries by thinking very creatively about problems. Furthermore, artists are often preoccupied with the technique of painting, and are concerned more with the materials they use than the pictures that they will eventually paint. The distinction between people who think and people who feel is very misleading. Everybody has thoughts, and everybody has feelings. In fact, the two are very closely related.

When we feel sad or happy, these feelings are often influenced by what we are thinking at the time. For example, if you sit down and bring to mind memories of a holiday that you really enjoyed, you will probably start to feel a little happier. On the other hand, if you sit down and try to remember a sad occasion, like a funeral, you will probably start to feel a little sadder. Although it is difficult to say exactly what's going on when we experience more complicated feelings like love, we can say that our thoughts are closely related to basic feelings like sadness and happiness. In fact, it is possible to suggest that thinking happy or sad thoughts can change our mood for better or for worse.

Negative thinking

We have already said that worriers tend to take a negative view of things. This is especially true when worriers view their own personalities. If you look at the worry items shown in Chapter 1 (Table 1.2), you will see that many of them reflect low levels of self-confidence. It is difficult to say why worriers take this dim view of the world and their own personal worth. Perhaps it could be that worry makes people think negatively, or it could be that thinking negatively makes people worry – the proverbial chicken and egg situation. It isn't easy to say which came first! For example, perhaps too much worry causes feelings of hopelessness. If you are always worrying about bad outcomes, then the future will always look bleak. It is difficult to think positively about yourself when you feel that you have nothing good to look forward to. On the other hand, if you are feeling 'down', then small problems will probably seem larger than they really are. Trivial events might be viewed as major catastrophes, triggering worry unnecessarily. In other words, the alarm system is constantly going off when there's nothing to be alarmed about. Although we don't know exactly why worrying and negative thinking appear in the same people, for our purposes such an answer is only of academic interest. As we said earlier, this chapter is about disarming thoughts that might cause us to abandon our coping efforts. It doesn't really matter why those thoughts occur.

It would appear that negative thinking has a powerful effect on mood. When people have difficulty coping, thoughts like 'I'm worthless' or 'I'm useless' pop into their minds automatically. If you do anything for long enough it will become automatic. For example, most people don't have to think about changing gear when they are driving. They simply do it automatically. When people get into the habit of thinking negatively about themselves, they do so with the same degree of automation. Derogatory remarks come to mind so easily that half the time they don't even realize what they're thinking. They feel sad, but don't see the connection between their thoughts and the way they feel.

However, psychologists and psychiatrists have found that these thoughts can be changed. Once an individual becomes aware of how thoughts can influence feelings, then he or she can learn to identify negative thoughts. Once negative thoughts have been identified, it is then possible to practise replacing them with more appropriate thoughts. This kind of treatment has become known as *cognitive therapy* or *cognitive behavioural therapy*, and is extremely helpful to those suffering from depression. Results show that cognitive therapy makes people less inclined to take a negative view of things, and therefore more able to deal with their problems.

At this point you might ask the question: 'Why should you replace negative thoughts if they are accurate?' The answer is, you shouldn't. A realistic evaluation of a problem may well be negative. However, psychologists have shown that people who think negatively are generally anything but realistic. The thoughts that they have are biased in favour of a negative view. In addition, negative thoughts are often treated mistakenly as facts. Negative thinkers rarely consider how accurate their automatic thoughts are. Most negative thoughts should be treated not as facts, but as possible facts that have to be tested. When we get a negative thought we should ask ourselves, 'Is this really true?' That way, we can discriminate between negative thoughts that reflect an accurate view of things and negative thoughts that are misleading. The process of self-questioning is very important. Usually, we don't believe everything we're told. If we did, then we could all be easily misled by the tabloids into believing, for example, that Elvis Presley is currently alive and well in Grimsby, and Second World War bombers can be found on the moon! Unfortunately, most people look at their own thoughts less critically than they do the Sunday papers. Sometimes our own thoughts are equally absurd! During cognitive therapy, most people are surprised to find that a little time spent challenging negative thoughts will reveal dramatic inaccuracies.

Earlier it was said that negative thoughts can be replaced with more appropriate thoughts – i.e. more *realistic*, not necessarily more 'positive', thoughts. So-called 'positive thinking' can be as unhelpful as negative thinking. It often involves replacing one unrealistic thought with a different kind of unrealistic thought. If you keep saying to yourself, 'Everything will be all right', when there is no good reason to think that things *will* be all right, then such a thought will be entirely inappropriate. Attempting to 'look on the bright side' when things are going wrong all around you will do you no good at all. Negative thoughts must always be replaced with realistic thoughts. The good news is that most realistic thoughts are more optimistic than negative thoughts, and considerably less rigid. Although a realistic thought acknowledges the negative side of things, it also acknowledges the possibility of things going well. For example, one might realistically say that 'Although I didn't do well today, I can always have another go tomorrow.' This is far more realistic than the negative thought, 'I didn't do well today, so I will never do well!'

For instance, you might have the thought, 'Nobody likes me' very often. Whenever you get this thought it probably makes you sad because whenever you get it you treat it as though it is a proven fact. If you were to examine your life more closely, you might see that not only do your family like you but also so do several people at work. Negative thoughts have to be carefully evaluated. They are often automatic and, because of this, wrong. However, because we treat them as facts, they can make us feel bad about ourselves and the world we live in.

Negative thinking and problem-solving

A negative style of thinking can be a handicap when trying to learn a new skill. As suggested earlier, you are bound to make some mistakes when attempting to problem-solve for the first time. If you consider these early attempts as 'failures', then you are more likely to give up. Of course, 'failures' can be a great disappointment. However, if you abandon your efforts too early, you are not allowing yourself the chance to improve your skills by frequent practice. Make a clear distinction in your mind between setbacks and failures. If you cannot solve a particular problem, then must you call your attempt 'a failure'? It would be more useful to see early difficulties as 'a temporary setback' – then you are more likely to renew your efforts. The word 'setback' is less final than 'failure'. Try to use it more often. After a setback, you may find that the next coping strategy you choose will work really well.

It is extremely common to confuse setbacks and failures. Binge-eating is a perfect example of how a setback, once viewed as a failure, can have unfortunate consequences. Let's consider Cathy and Liz.

Cathy

Cathy had been dieting for two weeks successfully and had lost 1.8 kg (4 lb). One evening, after a particularly stressful day at work, she started to get 'cravings' for chocolate. Cathy looked in her kitchen cupboard and found a packet of chocolate biscuits. After eating one, she felt very guilty. She began to have negative thoughts, like 'You'll never be able to diet' and 'You've blown it now.' Because Cathy considered her diet as a 'failed diet', it was, as far as she was concerned, over. She ate one biscuit after another without enjoying a single bite. In the morning she had a large breakfast, and within a fortnight she had put back the 1.8 kg she had lost.

Compare Cathy with Liz.

Liz

Liz had been successfully dieting for two weeks, and had also lost 1.8 kg. To relieve the boredom at work, she ate a bar of chocolate. Although Liz didn't feel good about breaking her diet, she also didn't feel that bad about it. She realized that a minor setback was no reason to abandon her diet altogether. As far as she was concerned, the fight was still on! 'Oh well,' Liz thought, 'It'll probably take me an extra day or two to get down to 56 kg (9 stone). So what!'

Clearly Liz has a more useful thinking style than Cathy. Not only are Liz's thoughts more helpful, they are also more realistic. If you break a diet it doesn't mean that the diet has failed at all. You can always have another go. Whenever you feel that you have 'failed' at something, remind yourself that this is most probably an unrealistic assessment of the situation. To say that you have experienced a setback is a much better description. Even if your setback is a considerable one, by seeing it as a 'setback' you are allowing yourself the chance to regain your position, given time.

In our example, Cathy doesn't question her thoughts. Because they are accepted as true statements, they have a profound effect on her behaviour. If you are like Cathy, then you may find that your attempts at problem-solving are prematurely abandoned because of negative thoughts. You must learn to recognize your negative thoughts, so that they can be replaced by more realistic thoughts. Every time you get a negative thought, you must try to challenge it rationally. Fortunately, negative thoughts are not that difficult to detect. In addition they can conveniently be grouped under headings, and we can take an example of a particular type of negative thought which will share features common with other negative thoughts in that group.

In the next section we list five types of negative thought. A heading is given, and underneath it an example of that type of thinking. As this chapter is about coping with problem-solving setbacks, all our examples will be closely related to this theme. However, you might try to think of other examples. After each type of negative thinking is explained, ways of challenging these thoughts will be considered. Examples of realistic replacements are given, but these are not the only ones available. Again, you might try thinking up some of your own.

Black-and-white thinking
Example: If I can't do problem-solving perfectly, then I may as well give up!

A black-and-white thinker sees things in terms of 'all or nothing'. Something must be either all good or totally bad. Our example is typical of this thinking style. Problem-solving has to be accomplished to a high standard, or it's not worth bothering with. This style of thinking can also account for Cathy's binge. Cathy most probably abandoned her diet because she could only think in an all-or-nothing way. To Cathy, she was either on a diet or off a diet. Eating a chocolate biscuit meant that she was 'off' and had therefore 'failed'.

This type of thinking is highly unproductive. If you have unrealistic expectations then you are setting yourself up for 'failure'. It is impossible to solve problems perfectly after one or two attempts. There will always be something that could have been done better. Remember, progress depends on practice. Improvements may be very gradual, but these small improvements will add up over time. Perhaps you won't be able to detect any improvements over several weeks. Perhaps your improvements will only be detectable over a period of several months. So, don't expect too much, too soon.

You might say to yourself, 'But what's the point in solving half of a problem? I'll still have something to worry about.' However, the point is, you have successfully solved half of it. This means you have 50 per cent less to worry about, and with continued effort you will probably solve the problem altogether. Making a little progress really is better than none at all. As we have said before, problem-solving might not actually solve your problem, but maybe will get you a step closer to solving a problem. If you reject problem-solving because it doesn't 'deliver the goods' immediately, then you might fail to see how tackling your problem has in fact got you one step closer to a less worry-filled life.

If you tend to think in black-and-white terms, remember to challenge yourself. Is this type of negative thought true? If you can't do problem-solving perfectly, does it really mean there are no advantages? Why can't you get better at problem-solving gradually?

Perhaps you could prepare some statements that you can read whenever you find yourself indulging in black-and-white thinking. For example:

Although I didn't solve my problem very effectively, I did feel more in control of my worry.

or

Maybe I could have defined my problem more accurately. The fact is, I know where I'm going wrong now, and next time I'll be able to do it better.

Overgeneralization
Example: Problem-solving didn't work now, so why should it ever work?

Overgeneralization is drawing sweeping conclusions on the basis of a single event. We often do this by making false connections. For example, you might think that because you can't play tennis very well, you probably can't play squash very well either. In fact the two games are very different, and it's quite easy to be a good squash player without being good at tennis! Another way we can overgeneralize is by thinking that one poor performance predicts another. Although this can be true of some things – for example, if you can't play the trumpet today, then it is unlikely you will be able to play it tomorrow – it most certainly isn't true of all things. Although you might find it difficult to problem-solve today, this may not be true tomorrow. Everybody has off days. All sorts of things might reduce our efficiency. Perhaps you are feeling too tense. Perhaps you are too tired. Perhaps there's too much noise outside. The important thing to remember is that if something goes wrong once, it doesn't mean that it will *always* go wrong.

The world is full of examples of failures preceding successes. Have you ever listened to cars starting on a cold morning? The first turn of the ignition key will usually fail to start the car. Does that mean the car will never start? Of course not. After anything between two and twenty turns you will hear the engine ticking over. For the driver, persistent effort has paid off. He or she will be able to get to work on time. In other words, the first attempts at starting the car were setbacks, not failures.

If you think that you overgeneralize, then be prepared to challenge your thoughts. Is it really true that because you never did well at school, you will never be 'clever' enough to deal with your problems? Why should today's disappointments stop you from succeeding tomorrow? Are there any good reasons why you should think in this way?

You might find preparing replacement thoughts like the following helpful, if you overgeneralize:

> Problem-solving didn't work as well as I thought. Maybe I should relax and try again later.

or

> Just because things went wrong today doesn't mean they won't work out tomorrow.

Blaming yourself
Example: It all went wrong because of me!

When things go wrong we often blame ourselves. This is because sometimes it's the easiest thing to do. Human beings are always trying to work out why things happen. If something goes wrong and there isn't an obvious reason why, then we will look for someone to blame. If there isn't anybody around to blame, we are likely to blame ourselves.

This need to accuse is particularly evident in the newspapers, especially after a disaster. On 15 April 1989 many football fans were tragically killed while attempting to get into the stadium at Hillsborough, Sheffield. Needless to say, the tabloids were soon baying for blood. The papers were alive with accusations and counter-accusations. First it was the police's fault for mishandling the situation. Then it was the fault of the supporters for behaving like hooligans. Then it was the government's fault for doing nothing about safety standards. Regardless of whose fault it was, the example serves to show how people often try to explain complicated events by suggesting a single cause – that is, the 'fault' of a particular individual or group. In most cases it is usually extremely difficult to prove that someone is blameworthy. When something like a disaster occurs, this is usually because a number of small things have been adding up. The same applies to our personal lives. If something goes wrong, it might be because a whole series of events have been leading up to it. Most of these events will probably be out of our control. Therefore it is senseless to indulge in self-blame.

If you cannot problem-solve efficiently, don't leap to the conclusion that you are lazy or negligent. Of course, it is possible that you are being lazy and negligent! However, such an evaluation is likely to be incorrect if you are a negative thinker. It is more likely that you are blaming yourself for a setback because that is what you usually do. A closer examination of the circumstances that led up to your setback might reveal the effects of factors out of your control.

If you feel that you haven't been very good at problem-solving, then try to establish why. Maybe you haven't put much effort into it, but this lack of commitment might be because of some other problem. Maybe you've only just got over the flu or are feeling tired or premenstrual, in which case is it really your fault? If you make mistakes because you are upset, then ask yourself why you are upset. Perhaps somebody was rude to you this morning. Was that your fault? If you habitually blame yourself, then it is time to break the habit. A close look at your mistakes will most probably reveal that some causes have little, if anything, to do with you. You cannot accept the blame for things that you cannot do anything about.

We have said before that problem-solving involves using a collection of skills. If you get these skills wrong occasionally, you may need more practice. Getting the skills wrong is not the same as *being* wrong. When things go wrong, get out of the habit of calling yourself names like 'stupid' or 'useless'. It is important to preserve a sense of self-worth and self-respect. Even if you do make mistakes sometimes, that does not mean that you are a worthless person!

Try to replace your blaming thoughts with more constructive statements. For example:

It was impossible for me to have known that that would happen –
I did my best.

or

Just because things went wrong this time doesn't mean that I'm
stupid.

Predicting the future
Example: It's sure to go wrong!

We all make predictions all the time. Although you probably don't
think of it as predicting, every time you leave your house or flat to
go shopping you are in fact making several predictions. The most
important one is that the shops will be open. A second important prediction might be that the shops will have what you want
to buy. However, even simple predictions like this are sometimes
incorrect. We often find shops unexpectedly closed. Or perhaps
they have sold out of the commodities we require.

At best, we only ever have a rough idea of what is going to
happen in the future. Clearly, some things are more likely than
others. For example, it is more likely that you will buy magazines
more regularly than cars. However, there is no such thing as an
absolute certainty. Even things that seem impossible can actually
happen. In *Guinness World Records* is a man who has been struck by
lightning seven times! One would imagine that after being struck
once such a man might be excused developing a fairly relaxed attitude to storms. After all, the chances of being hit twice are ridicu-
lously small, aren't they?

If you are a negative thinker, then most of your predictions will
favour negative outcomes. In addition, you will have a tendency to
treat these negative predictions as facts. As we have already stressed
several times before, the future is uncertain. Although some things
are more likely than others, it is unlikely that everything will turn
out bad all the time! Such predictions are clearly biased.

If you have already predicted that 'problem-solving won't stop
you worrying', then challenge that prediction. How can you be so
sure? A more realistic prediction would be that 'problem-solving
may or may not stop me worrying'. This latter prediction is far

more realistic. It acknowledges the fact that you are not psychic and cannot look into the future! Also, unlike the former prediction, it recognizes the possibility of things turning out all right, as well as going wrong. Not only is it more realistic, it also avoids unnecessary pessimism.

Finally, a word should be said about 'mind-reading'. This is when we predict what other people are thinking, and how they will react. As with predicting the future, we know that some things are more likely than others. Our best friend is less likely to hit us than our worst enemy. However, we should never assume that we know what's going on in somebody else's head. If you have a tendency to think the worst, then always try to examine the evidence for and against your predictions. Some alternative thoughts that might replace your negative predictions are:

I keep thinking things won't work out – but in fact it's impossible to predict the future.

or

I keep on predicting how other people will react – but it's impossible to say, I'm not a mind-reader.

Dismissing successes
Example: I solved this problem, but so what!

Last of all, don't dismiss your successes. If you solve one problem, then good for you. That means you can solve another, and another after that. The more problems you solve, the less you will have to worry about. You can get out of the habit of dismissing your successes by rewarding yourself. We have already considered reward menus in Chapter 3, so we won't go over them again. Needless to say, if you succeed, reward yourself.

Remember, when you do solve a problem, it really does mean something. It means that you have taken control of your life. It means that you are less vulnerable to worry, and therefore less likely to suffer the consequences, like sleepless nights. In the long term, this means you will be a healthier, fitter person. When you manage to solve a problem, you will be able to concentrate more on the things you enjoy. Finally, it means that you will be better equipped the next time a problem develops in your life. Remind yourself that problem-solving is an achievement that deserves rewarding.

Perhaps you could prepare statements like the following:

Because I solved my problem, I haven't worried for a week. That's quite an achievement.

or

Well done! I solved the problem: I'll go to the cinema tonight as a reward.

The points we've been considering were examples of negative thinking styles, and the kind of thoughts that they generate. This kind of thinking can be very discouraging, and you might be tempted to give up problem-solving if you get these thoughts often. However, if you constantly challenge these thoughts and look for facts that disprove them, you will soon learn that negative thinking is not only unhelpful, but largely misleading. The future is not always as bleak as you might think.

6

When the worry won't stop

This is not a pessimistic final chapter. Although we will acknowledge that sometimes worry can't be stopped, we will also try to establish reasons why this might happen. We will be approaching this difficulty in much the same way as we have approached every other difficulty – systematically and with the intention of coping successfully. This chapter represents an extension of the techniques we have already learned. We will again be defining the problem, working out ways of dealing with it, and choosing an appropriate set of coping strategies. However, these coping strategies will be, now and again, a little different from those described earlier.

So, let us define the problem. You are worried. You have used the techniques described in this book to problem-solve, and you find that you still can't stop worrying. Why should this happen? We can suggest three reasons. First, it may be that you still haven't 'got the hang' of problem-solving and more practice is required. Second, it may be that your problem cannot be solved. Although this is quite rare, most people will at one time or another be forced to admit that a situation or circumstance is simply uncontrollable. However, there are ways of dealing with 'insoluble' problems. We will be considering some of these in a moment. Finally, if you can't stop worrying, it could be that your worries are part of a more complicated emotional problem. For example, certain types of anxiety disorder are associated with excessive worry, and this kind of worry is quite difficult to stop on your own. For our purposes, we can consider worry as a component of anxiety. 'Worry' is a specific term, whereas 'anxiety' is a more general term. The experience of anxiety can be broken down into three parts: behaviours, physical changes and unpleasant thoughts. So, when people become anxious they will change their behaviour, notice that their body 'feels' different and worry more. For example, a spider-phobic might run out of the bathroom when he sees a spider in the bath. This is a change of behaviour. He will also be reluctant to go back into the bathroom; one might say that he is trying to 'avoid' the spider. Further, he will know that he is anxious because his body will feel different. His heart rate might increase, his mouth might go dry, he might begin to sweat. Finally, he might experience unpleasant thoughts like 'That spider was so big it will be able to get out of the bath. It might crawl into the bedroom while I'm asleep.' These unpleasant thoughts are really worries. He is anticipating an upsetting event. Specific phobias, like a fear of insects or dogs, are not strongly associated with worry, but more with behavioural changes. However, there are some anxiety problems where worry plays a more significant role. We will give this matter further consideration shortly.

In the following section we will deal with the first of these reasons why worry won't stop.

What to do if you still need more practice!

Let's assume that although you have been trying to problem-solve regularly, your efforts have been unsuccessful. For the sake of making the difficulty explicit, let's say that when trying to define a problem, you are always unable to trace the worry back to a single cause. This results in the section of inappropriate coping strategies and continued worry. What can be done under these circumstances?

First of all, you could remind yourself that practice will eventually improve your problem-solving skills. Although you find problem definition hard today, this might not be the case tomorrow. Second, you could strengthen your resolve to succeed by 'inoculating' yourself against negative thinking. Reconsider the information in Chapter 5. Remind yourself of the distinction between setbacks and failure, and then identify any negative thoughts you might have experienced. If you notice that you have been 'overgeneralizing' or perhaps 'predicting the future', then challenge these thoughts and replace them with more realistic thoughts. Finally, when you are in a relaxed frame of mind, have another go at defining the problem.

Although the above suggestions might help you to cope with a temporary setback, they do not reduce the impact of your existing problem or problems. You are still worrying, and as yet are unsure if your next attempt at problem-solving will have the desired effect. Under these circumstances, what can you do?

First of all, recognize that worry is 'catastrophic'. If you have been worrying a great deal, then it is quite possible that the 'disasters' you anticipate will never actually happen. Look at the worry questionnaire in Chapter 1 (Table 1.2). You will probably be able to identify a group of concerns, or maybe a particular worry that you have had in the past. Consider the five main worry areas again: relationships, lack of confidence, an aimless future, work incompetence and financial problems. Now, ask yourself the following questions:

• How many people do I know who have been unable to survive a relationship problem?
• How many people do I know who simply couldn't cope with life because they lacked confidence?
• How many people do I know who have never achieved a single ambition?
• How many people do I know who have lost their jobs because they made too many mistakes?
• Finally, how many people do I know who have found themselves in serious trouble – for example, prison – because of financial problems?

Unless you have an extremely unlucky group of friends, the answer to most if not all of the above questions will be few or none! The worst very rarely happens. Even if we can't solve our problems, unpleasant consequences are rarely as catastrophic as we imagine. Coping with a real bad outcome is sometimes easier than coping with an imagined one. If you can't solve your problems yet, then remind yourself that worry can turn molehills into mountains. When the 'disaster' arrives, you might be surprised to find how inconsequential the effects are. We are not suggesting here that terrible things don't happen. This would be untrue. However, we must balance this acknowledgement with a realistic appreciation of how unlikely terrible things are. A single life is not long enough to contain the number of potential disasters most worriers anticipate! Financial worries provide us with a good example of how an anticipated catastrophe is often found to be, in the event, nothing more than an irritating inconvenience. Below, the phenomenon of credit card debt will be considered in some detail.

Given the 'mindbending' power of advertising, it's not surprising that most of us give in to consumer pressure. We are made to feel that our lives won't be worth living unless we purchase the latest clothes, music or gadget. Because of this, 'money worries' are fairly high on everybody's agenda. It would be difficult to find somebody who had never got into debt! Most of us know what it's like to enjoy spending the bank's money without considering how we're going to pay it back.

The average credit card debt for families with a reasonable income is around £3,200, while average overall debt per household, including overdrafts and personal loans, is between £6,000 and £8,000. Such a debt often causes arguments, bad feelings and sleepless nights. Although this is a large sum of money, we must ask ourselves: what happens to most families who overspend? Do the bailiffs arrive in the small hours, waving a repossession order? Do nightmares of destitution and poverty become a sad reality?

Although this *can* happen, it very rarely does. In fact, it happens with remarkable infrequency given the number of people who overspend! Under normal circumstances, the consequences of overspending are less dramatic. People are usually forced to negotiate repayment at a different rate. As a consequence of this, a holiday might need to be cancelled, or some leisure activities given up. In other words, getting out of debt involves having to forgo a number of pleasures, until the debt is paid off or reduced to a more manageable level.

The important thing to remember is that although people agonize over their debts, the consequences are almost always less catastrophic than those anticipated while worrying. If one considers the consequences of financial problems in some of the poorest countries, this gives us a measure of how unwarranted our financial worries are. Even if we have a £1,500 credit card debt, this will not mean for most of us starvation and homelessness!

So, let's summarize. If you're finding it difficult to problem-solve, then remind yourself that more effort will probably be a worthwhile investment. Second, remind yourself that worry is catastrophic. Most of the disasters that you imagine simply won't happen. Finally, remember that even if the worst does happen, the consequences might not be as terrible as you anticipate.

Problems that can't be solved

Some things that make us worry we can do nothing about. Even if we are efficient problem-solvers, situations occur that we cannot change. This kind of 'insoluble' problem is quite different from the 'insoluble' problems discussed in the last section. A problem that can be solved by perseverance is somehow less daunting than a problem that appears totally resistant to resolution. When we know that we can't solve a problem whatever we do, this can be quite depressing. We feel that we cannot exercise any control over our lives.

Ageing and dying are two obvious examples of insoluble problems. Although we can choose to eat nutritious foods instead of junk foods, and choose exercise instead of inactivity, these measures can only provide a partially successful 'solution' to the problems of age and death. A healthy lifestyle might retard ageing and allow us to see our grandchildren grow up, but we must still face the fact that old age and death are inescapable.

Not all insoluble problems are as dramatic as ageing and dying. For example, psychologists and psychiatrists have found that it is very difficult to stop people being jealous. Although there have been many attempts to solve the problem of jealousy, a recent review of treatments suggests that little can be done. Becoming vulnerable to jealousy appears to be one of the inevitable costs of falling in love. Another common example of an 'insoluble' problem is physical illness. Once you become ill, there isn't a lot you can do about it. You might be able to take some medicine, but this will take effect in its own time.

In addition to the above it is interesting to note that people often report worrying quite a lot about social and political problems. Although these can be solved by the slow process of political change, there are few things that the individual can do to speed things up. Voting in a general election, signing petitions and protesting will have some effect, but desired changes will not happen overnight. Further, the threat of terrorism, starvation in the Global South and climate change will be with us for some time to come.

So, not every problem is readily solved. Let's remind ourselves what sort of problem we're considering here. Getting older, and coming to terms with the fact that we will one day die are two dramatic sources of worry. We cannot make the clock go backwards. Similarly, disease and illnesses continue according to biological processes, which may or may not respond to medication or surgery. Although we can try as hard as we can to follow 'doctor's orders', our influence over the progress of some illnesses is very limited. Finally, the social and political problems of the world are largely resistant to our protests and complaints. Although we might see that many of the world's problems could be 'solved' overnight, the fact is they won't be. Political changes – especially those requiring cooperation between different countries – can be a long time coming. But we can stop treating the world as a problem, and treat our emotions as a problem instead. Even when we face inevitabilities, we are not totally powerless We can still try to change ourselves.

This distinction between changing the world and changing our *response* to the world is an important one. Psychologists have called these two ways of coping *problem-focused coping* and *emotion-focused coping*. Problem-focused coping is what happens when you tackle the problem at source. Most of the examples in this book describe people using problem-focused coping. In Chapter 4, Jo decided that she would save her relationship by seeing a counsellor; Andrew addressed his social anxiety by improving his conversational skills; and Jane was able to cope with a difficult meeting by working harder. In all these examples, our characters could change their circumstances by doing something different.

When doing something different will have no effect on the problem, then it is best to endorse an emotion-focused coping strategy. Instead of attempting to change the world, you must attempt to change the way you are reacting to the world. For example, although you cannot do anything about an illness, you can still try to alter the way you feel about it. If you are frightened, you might try to turn that fear into peaceful resignation. When we worry, we are responding to an anticipated threat. If we can change the way we feel about a particular threat, be it an illness, getting old or anything else over which we have no direct control, we might worry about it less.

When you find that problem-solving isn't working, then reconsider the nature of your problem. Can you really do anything about it? The answer to this question is extremely important. If you decide you can do something about it when in fact you can't, then you may find yourself 'banging your head against a brick wall'. Attempting to solve an insoluble problem can be upsetting and frustrating. If you are worrying over a problem that you cannot seem to solve, then re-evaluate your approach. Perhaps problem-focused coping should be abandoned in favour of emotion-focused coping. Remember, we are not abandoning problem-solving.

Emotion-focused coping is simply a different sort of problem-solving, in which the problem is defined in terms of an emotional reaction. How then might we change our emotional responses? We will answer this question next.

The relationship between the individual and his or her emotions is a complicated one. Therefore, it would be misleading to suggest that changing our emotional response is easy. We must consider not only the intensity of an emotional reaction, but also the strengths and weaknesses of the person dealing with that reaction.

If the cause of worry is a problem that might have very upsetting consequences, then sometimes the best thing to do is to avoid thinking about that problem. Psychologists call this reaction 'denial'. It can be very effective. Indeed, there is evidence to suggest that some people suffering from very serious illnesses fare better when they are able to 'deny' their problem. In addition, recent research has shown that people who have experienced really terrible things in the past – such as concentration camps – are able to lead happier lives if they ignore their bad thoughts.

If you know that something very upsetting is going to happen, then try to distract yourself when you become apprehensive. As we have suggested earlier, you may find watching a film can take your mind off things. On the other hand, seeing friends or relatives may be more useful to you.

Of course, learning to ignore bad thoughts isn't easy. Not everybody can develop this skill. The situation is complicated further by the results of experiments which show that trying to suppress thoughts can result in their more frequent return. In this kind of experiment people are given a word, or image, and told not to think about it. After a short while, they are told that they can think of whatever they like. People who have been trying to avoid thinking about a particular word or image find that it comes back more than if they had never suppressed it in the first place!

Given that everybody is different, the only sensible thing to do is to conduct an experiment using yourself as a guinea-pig. Try denial and see if it works for you. If ignoring your bad thoughts makes life easier, then try to improve this skill. If you find that it makes matters worse, then obviously it would be foolish to continue using this strategy.

If your problem is only moderately upsetting, then confronting your fears, rather than avoiding them, will probably be more useful. In Chapter 1 we briefly mentioned exposure therapies. Psychologists often treat fears by exposing people directly to what it is that they're frightened of. For example, a person suffering from agoraphobia (a fear of going out of the house) might be encouraged to walk down to the shops. After staying outside for a long period of time, the agoraphobic might become adjusted to being outside, and experience a reduction in fear.

If you are worried about some unavoidable problem, then provided the outcome is not too distressing facing that problem might be the best way to deal with it. You can face an unavoidable problem by thinking about it yourself, or perhaps talking over implications with other people. A friend's voice, the touch of another's hand or an expression of affection can provide much needed support in these circumstances. It's always easier to face a problem if you can share your feelings about it with someone else. Try to be honest. Don't keep your feelings bottled up or try to put on a 'brave' face. If you want to cry, then go ahead and cry. If you're frightened, then say so. In this way, you will be able to get a clear view of how you are feeling. Sometimes it is necessary to 'let things out', if change is to take place.

By exploring your worries and concerns, you will be subjecting yourself to an experience closely related to therapeutic exposure. Hopefully, continued exposure will result in a step-by-step reduction in your levels of fear and apprehension.

So far we have suggested that both avoiding and facing your problems may be useful, depending on what sort of person you are and how serious the problem is. However, it might be the case that both these techniques can be used together. If you are upset or tired, then bad thoughts might best be ignored. If you can only do this for a short time, then this may be all that's needed. A few hours later you might be feeling more relaxed and ready to face your problem. If ignoring your bad thoughts makes them return with greater frequency, then this will not matter so much. After all, you are only delaying the process of dealing with them for a short while.

Worry and anxiety

Sometimes worry can be part of a more serious problem. For example, when people get extremely anxious, worries become vivid and particularly difficult to control. If these worries become too intrusive, then an anxious person might need to seek help. When health professionals talk about anxiety, they are not talking about a single problem. In fact, there are a whole group of problems which are related in some way to the experience of anxiety. For example, phobias, sudden panics and obsessions are all described as anxiety problems.

Clearly, a thorough examination of anxiety problems is beyond the scope of this book. However, if you want to know more about anxiety, a number of books dealing with the topic are currently available. These books usually describe the symptoms of anxiety and provide valuable information on self-help. Because this book is about common worry, we will not attempt to detail this kind of information here but you will find examples of these books in 'Further reading'. However, we shall briefly consider one example of an anxiety problem: *generalized anxiety disorder (GAD)*. Generalized anxiety, sometimes also described as 'free-floating anxiety', is suitable for consideration in this book, because it is a problem strongly associated with worry.

People who suffer from generalized anxiety are usually very tense, and worry excessively. Sweating, flushing, a pounding heart and 'upset stomach' are frequently experienced, often accompanied by worries about losing control in a public place, having a heart attack or becoming fatally ill.

These symptoms – upsetting thoughts and unpleasant bodily sensations – can appear without any apparent cause. Because these symptoms are sometimes difficult to account for, the anxious person is often treated unsympathetically at home. Many people suffering from generalized anxiety are perfectly aware that many of their worries appear strange to other people. However, this recognition has no effect on the amount of worry experienced. Misfortunes continue to be anticipated even if they never actually happen.

If generalized anxiety becomes too difficult to live with, then it is advisable to seek help. This usually means a visit to the family doctor, who may recommend talking therapies such as counselling or cognitive behavioural therapy (CBT). CBT helps you identify unhelpful and unrealistic beliefs and behaviour, and replace them with more helpful and realistic ones. Effective relaxation techniques may also be suggested. Your GP can also offer medication. The options should be discussed in detail and, depending on your symptoms, include selective serotonin reuptake inhibitors (SSRIs), antidepressants that increase the level of the chemical serotonin in your brain, and sometimes, as a short-term measure, tranquillizers, usually one of a group of drugs called the benzodiazepines. Although tranquillizers can be helpful in the short term, they are usually unhelpful and definitely addictive if taken for an extended period of time. A number of side effects are associated with tranquillizers, including severe headaches and nausea. However, the most serious problem by far with benzodiazepines is that they are addictive, and this can be both distressing in itself and difficult to overcome. For this reason, the National Institute for Health and Care Excellence (NICE) strongly advises against their use except in crisis, while the Royal College of GPs also advises great care in prescribing such drugs.. An estimated 1.5 million people in the UK are addicted to benzodiazepines, often older people as a result of over-prescribing decades ago. (To find out more about prescription medication addiction, read *Tranquillizers and Antidepressants: When to take them, how to stop* by Professor Malcolm Lader (Sheldon Press, 2008).)

Ideally, a general practitioner will refer anxiety patients through the NHS for treatment with a clinical psychologist. Most clinical psychologists help people to manage their worries and anxiety by using something called *anxiety management training*, which usually involves learning about relaxation, discussing worries in some detail, and also learning to face particular situations if you find that they are associated with increased levels of anxiety. Anxiety management training can be given to individual patients, or to patients attending a clinic in small groups. If you think that you are suffering from generalized anxiety and think you might have to see a clinical psychologist, remember: this does not mean that you are mad, mentally ill or sick. Because you are not suffering from a disease or illness you will not receive drugs or medication.

Clinical psychologists tend to treat anxiety as a normal emotional response. After all, it can be very useful. If you climb to the top of a ladder, you will probably experience some mild anxiety. This alerts you to the potential danger of falling off and you exercise appropriate caution; if you were totally relaxed in this situation, then you might stop taking care. Clearly, this would increase your chances of having a serious accident. Psychologists don't try to get rid of anxiety, because anxiety is a normal emotional response, but only attempt to reduce levels of anxiety so that life can go on without unnecessary disruptions.

Conclusions

In this chapter we have considered worries that cannot be dealt with by problem-solving. However, let us end on an optimistic note. There are few problems that you will be able to do nothing about. If you are having trouble dealing with problems because you need more practice at problem-solving, then it will only be a matter of time before your skills improve to the extent that worry is reduced. If your problem is genuinely 'insoluble', then we have mentioned the idea of emotion-focused coping. Although you might not be able to solve the problem that's making you worry, you might be able to change the way you feel about it. If this change is successful, you will probably worry less. Finally, although you may find worry difficult to deal with if it is part of an anxiety problem, that does not mean that you will never be able to deal with it. If you see a clinical psychologist, then you will be taught a number of skills that will help you to reduce levels of anxiety and the amount you worry.

The circumstances outlined above are exceptional. Virtually all the worries you are likely to have will be related to everyday life problems, which can be solved using problem-solving techniques. By systematically analysing your problems, you will be able to generate solutions capable of resolving them. Armed with a systematic approach, you will be able to use worry constructively. Hopefully, after reading this book, you will see worry as helpful rather than harmful!

Further reading

If you are a health professional then you will no doubt be aware that relatively little research has been conducted into the subject of worry, compared to research in other anxiety disorders. Given the ubiquity of worry, it is remarkable how little attention the phenomenon has commanded in the clinical literature. It has been suggested that this neglect has been due to inadequate definition; the considerable overlap between worry and anxiety may well have retarded the development of 'worry' as a discrete concept worthy of closer scrutiny. However, even excepting adequate definition, the term continues to be used – for example, in the *Diagnostic and Statistical Manual* of the American Psychiatric Association – and the increasing incidence of worry in normal populations noted. Further, the importance of involuntary cognitive activity in psychological disorders is now widely recognized.

Consideration of historical factors might also suggest reasons for this neglect of worry in the literature. The concept is associated with clinical practice, and may have escaped scientific attention through the influence of traditional behaviourism. The investigation of 'internal' phenomena in clinical populations is a relatively recent development, largely due to the ascent and expansion of modern cognitive psychology. It would seem reasonable to suggest that worry has had to wait for the convergence of two historically independent traditions to capture academic interest. The following reading list may be of some interest and practical use:

Andrea, H., Beurskens, A. J. H. M., Kant, I. J., Davey, G. C. L., Field, A. P. and van Schayck, C. P. (2004) 'The relation between pathological worrying and fatigue in a working population', *Journal of Psychosomatic Research*, 57 (4), 399–407.

Behar, E., Alcaine, O., Zuellig, A. R. and Borkovec, T. D. (2003) 'Screening for generalized anxiety disorder using the Penn State Worry Questionnaire: a receiver operating characteristics analysis', *Journal of Behavior Therapy and Experimental Psychiatry*, 34, 25–43.

Borkovec, T. D., Robinson, E., Pruzinsky, T. and DePree, J. A. (1983) 'Preliminary exploration of worry: some characteristics and processes', *Behavior, Research, and Therapy*, 21, 9–12.

Borkovec, T. D., Wilkinson, L., Folensbee, R. and Lerman, C. (1983) 'Stimulus control applications to the treatment of worry', *Behavior, Research, and Therapy*, 21, 247–51.

Borkovec T. D., Metzger R. L. and Pruzinsky T. (1986) 'Anxiety, worry, and the self', in L. Hartman and K. R. Blankstein (eds) *Perception of Self in Emotional Disorder and Psychotherapy*, New York: Plenum Publishers.

Borkovec, T. D., Alcaine, O. and Behar, E. (2004) 'Avoidance theory of worry and generalized anxiety disorder', in R. G. Heimberg, C. L. Turk and D. S. Mennin (eds) *Generalized Anxiety Disorder: Advances in research and practice* (pp. 77–108), New York: Guilford Press.

Breznitz, S. (1971) 'A study of worrying', *British Journal of Social and Clinical Psychology*, 10, 271–9.

Brosschot, J. F., Gerin, W. and Thayer, J. F. (2006) 'The perseverative cognition hypothesis: a review of worry, prolonged stress-related physiological activation, and health', *Journal of Psychosomatic Research*, 60 (2), 113–24.

Dash, S. R., Meeten, F., Jones, F. and Davey, G. C. L. (2013) 'Socialisation to the mood-as-input model as a method for reducing worry', manuscript in preparation.

Davey, G. C. L. and Wells, A. (2006) *Worry and its Psychological Disorders: Theory, assessment, and treatment*, Chichester: John Wiley & Sons.

Deffenbacher, J. L. (1980) 'Worry and emotionality in test anxiety', in I. G. Sarason (ed.) *Test Anxiety: Theory, research and applications* (pp. 111–28), Hillsdale, New Jersey: Lawrence Erlbaum Associates.

Eysenck, M. W. (1984) 'Anxiety and the worry process', *Bulletin of the Psychonomic Society*, 22, 545–8.

Meeten, F. and Davey, G. C. L. (2011) 'Mood-as-input hypothesis and perseverative psychopathologies', *Clinical Psychology Review*, 31, 1259–75.

Mohlman, K. et al. (2009) 'The relation of worry to prefrontal cortex volume in older adults with and without generalized anxiety disorder', *Psychiatry Research: Neuroimaging*, 173 (2), 121–7.

Newman, M. G. and Borkovec, T. D. (1995) 'Cognitive-behavioral treatment of generalized anxiety disorder', *The Clinical Psychologist*, 48 (4), 5–7.

Nuevo, R., Montorio, I. and Borkovec, T. D. (2004) 'A test of the role of meta-worry in the prediction of worry severity in an elderly sample', *Journal of Behavior Therapy and Experimental Psychiatry*, 35, 209–19.

Ruscio, A. and Borkovec, T. D. (2004) 'Experience and appraisal of worry among high worriers with and without generalized anxiety disorder', *Behaviour Research and Therapy*, 42 (12), 469–82.

Smith, J. M. and Alloy, L. B. (2009) 'A roadmap to rumination: a review of the definition, assessment, and conceptualization of this multifaceted construct', *Clinical Psychology Review*, 29 (2), 116–28.

Stöber, J. and Borkovec, T. D. (2002) 'Reduced concreteness of worry in generalized anxiety disorder: findings from a therapy study', *Cognitive Therapy and Research*, 26, 89–96.

Tallis, F. (1989) 'Worry: a cognitive analysis', unpublished doctoral dissertation, University of London.

Tallis, F. and Eysenck, M. W. (1994) 'Worry: mechanisms and modulating influences', *Behavioural and Cognitive Psychotherapy*, 22 (1), 37–56.

Books on anxiety (see p. 73)

Barlow, D. (2004) *Anxiety and Its Disorders: The nature and treatment of anxiety and panic*, New York: Guilford Press.

Foreman, E. I. et al. (new edition, 2007) *Overcoming Anxiety for Dummies*, Chichester: John Wiley & Sons.

Kennerley, H. (2009) *Overcoming Anxiety: A self-help guide using cognitive behavioral techniques*, London: Constable & Robinson.

Marks, I. M. (second edition, 2005) *Learning to Live with Fear: Understanding and coping with anxiety*, New York: McGraw Hill Professional.

Shafran, R. et al. (2013) *The Complete CBT Guide for Anxiety: A self-help guide for anxiety, panic, social anxiety, phobias, health anxiety and obsessive compulsive disorder*, London: Constable & Robinson.

Toates, F. and Coschug-Toates, O. (second edition, 2002) *Obsessive Compulsive Disorder*, London: Class Publishing.

In addition, for those who are already anxious and taking benzodiazepines, and who would like to stop:

Lader, M. (2008) *Tranquillizers and Antidepressants: When to take them, how to stop*, London: Sheldon Press.

Index